Psychological and Psychiatric Issues in Patients With Chronic Pain

What Do I Do Now? – Pain Medicine

Mark P. Jensen and Lynn R. Webster
Series Editors

PUBLISHED AND FORTHCOMING TITLES:

*Psychiatric and Psychological Issues in Patients with
    Chronic Pain* by Daniel M. Doleys
Painful Conditions of the Upper Limb by Ramon Cuevas
Headache by Olivia Begasse de Dhaem and Carolyn A. Bernstein
Neuropathic Pain by Nadine Attal and Didier Bouhassira
Management of Sickle Cell Pain by Wally R. Smith and Thokozeni Lipato

Psychological and Psychiatric Issues in Patients With Chronic Pain

Daniel M. Doleys, PhD
Director, Doleys Clinic/Pain and Rehabilitation Institute

With Contributions by Nicholas D. Doleys

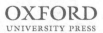
OXFORD
UNIVERSITY PRESS

OXFORD
UNIVERSITY PRESS

Oxford University Press is a department of the University of Oxford. It furthers
the University's objective of excellence in research, scholarship, and education
by publishing worldwide. Oxford is a registered trade mark of Oxford University
Press in the UK and certain other countries.

Published in the United States of America by Oxford University Press
198 Madison Avenue, New York, NY 10016, United States of America.

Library of Congress Cataloging-in-Publication Data
Names: Doleys, Daniel M., author. | Doleys, Nicholas D., author.
Title: Psychological and Psychiatric Issues in Patients with Chronic Pain /
Daniel M. Doleys ; with contributions by Nicholas D. Doleys.
Description: New York, NY : Oxford University Press, [2021] |
Includes bibliographical references and index.
Identifiers: LCCN 2020047164 (print) | LCCN 2020047165 (ebook) |
ISBN 9780197544631 (paperback) | ISBN 9780197544655 (epub) |
ISBN 9780197544662 (online)
Subjects: MESH: Chronic Pain—psychology | Chronic Pain—therapy |
Pain Management—psychology | Case Reports
Classification: LCC RB127.5.C48 (print) | LCC RB127.5.C48 (ebook) |
NLM WL 704 | DDC 616/.0472—dc23
LC record available at https://lccn.loc.gov/2020047164
LC ebook record available at https://lccn.loc.gov/2020047165

DOI: 10.1093/med/9780197544631.001.0001

9 8 7 6 5 4 3 2 1

Printed by Marquis, Canada

To the patients suffering from chronic pain, their families/significant others, and especially the clinicians who care for them. DMD

To my sons, Dawson Parker and Shepard Henry. NDD

Contents

Scope and Complexities of the Clinical Issues 1

SECTION 1: CASE STUDIES

1 **A Broken Life** 9

2 **Haunted by Pain, Fatigue, and Insomnia** 17

3 **The Hand That Wouldn't Move** 27

4 **Something Doesn't Seem Right** 35

5 **How Many More Are There?** 43

6 **How Can Someone Do This to Themselves?** 51

7 **An All-Consuming Problem** 61

8 **Psychologically Immobilized and Functionally Paralyzed** 71

9 **The "What If" and "Yes But" Syndrome** 79

10 **The Patient Who Remembers Tomorrow** 87

11 **Please, Find It and Fix It** 97

12 **The Unseen Reality** 107

13 **There Are Not Enough Sheep** 117

14 **The Easy but Harmful Solution** 127

15 **Is This All There Is?** 135

16 **No Way That's My Drug Screen** 147

17 **The Abandoned Patient** 157

18 **The Not-So-Perfect Remedy** 165

19 **Teenager With Disabling Leg Pain** 179

SECTION 2: GENERAL CONSIDERATIONS

20 **Psychogenic Pain: A Useful Concept?** 189

21 Psychological/Behavioral Therapies 211

22 The Psychology of Opioid Tapering 231

Index 251

Scope and Complexities of the Clinical Issues

The term "clinician" is used throughout this book, in the most generic sense. This book is intended for any professional regularly encountering patients with pain, especially chronic pain. It is mostly geared toward the medical provider, MD, DO, PA, and CRNP, especially those in the primary-care setting. It is obviously suitable to the psychologist and psychiatrist. Front-line healthcare providers (e.g., nurses, physical therapists, and occupational therapists) will also find the book useful in their practice.

This book places a heavy emphasis on the context in which the problem exist. In this sense, it is a bit of a throwback to Sir William Osler's assertions, "It is much more important to know what sort of patient has the disease, than what sort of disease the patient has" and "The good physician treats the disease; the great physician treats the patient who has the disease." This book also acknowledges the complexity of the clinician–patient interaction, which has been aptly described as an event when the observer and observed are "locked inextricably in a dance that defines the impossibility of objectivity" (Quintner et al, 2008, p. 828). Nonetheless, the clinician is called upon to make, and execute, a decision that is in the best interest of the patient—and that falls within generally acceptable standards of care.

There is no attempt to turn the reader into an amateur psychologist. At the same time, many clinicians will find knowledge regarding psychological principals and interventions useful in providing effective patient care. Also, in the case of chronic pain, and when considering the many factors that contribute to chronic pain, one is dealing with a problem having significant psychological overtones, existing in a psychological being. By its very nature, the office or clinic visit is a psychosocial event. So, it is not a matter of if psychological principles are applied, but whether it is done by design or haphazardly. The clinician's degree of psychological sophistication, intended or not, will impact the effectiveness of the therapy.

What *Do I Do Now* is not an academic book, but it does contain evidenced-based research. It is not a clinical book, but it does contain clinical suggestions and recommendations. More than anything else, it is designed to stimulate critical clinical thinking. *What Do I Do Now* is intended to be a pocket guide and not an encyclopedia. It is no secret that there are many approaches to clinical dilemmas that will never be subjected to randomized clinical trials. Much of what is done in the practice of pain medicine is, indeed, "off label" and reflects the "art" of pain medicine. Most clinicians are guided by basic principles rather than fixed algorithms. They have to be fast on their feet and prepared for the unexpected. Clinical acumen varies. Not every approach works for everyone one, nor does it work in the same way when it does work.

At one time or another, over the span of over forty years, the authors have encountered every case, diagnosis, and patient type presented. A significant group of patients have been followed for ten years or more; some for as much as twenty years. Cases such as delusional parasitosis and multiple personality disorder are admittedly rare. One might go their entire career without seeing such, or at least not recognizing the patient as such. They are included herein as a means of attempting to broaden the way we view pain, especially chronic pain.

The International Association for the Study of Pain's ("The Need of a Taxonomy," 1979) definition has been foundational and very heuristic but has been to the subject of some philosophical as well as epistemological debates (Aydede and Shriver, 2018). It may be overly ambitious to hope that any one definition would effectively cover all pain-related situations, ranging from the fetus to the elderly, especially in light of dealing with a subjective and contextual phenomenon. Unusual cases are often regarded as the exception to the rule, but they, indeed, may point to the need to clarify the rule. It is this complexity that makes pain unlike any other disease or illness.

Some of the suggestions provided in this book may seem unconventional. Some have emerged from clinical experience. Wherever possible, published research is cited to support a position or statement. However, there are occasions where the author's provides an experienced-based opinion. There is the occasional humorous anecdote or tongue-in-cheek comments; no offense is intend. A sense of humor helps to get one through the day. This can be a very difficult group of patients. Clinician burnout is often as much mental as physical.

This book is part of the What Do I Do Now?—Pain Medicine series and follows the format of that series. The Problems and Disorders section involves case presentation designed to be to the point. However, it does reflect actual patient scenarios. There is no particular purpose to the order of presentation. Each case presentation will (a) include background information to aid in the recognition of the problem, (b) promote understating the problem within a broad context-biopsychosocial model, and (c) encourage the application of a measure of empathy to the decision making process.

This book recognizes that most clinicians in the primary care setting do not always have the time or resources to conduct the type of assessment that each case may require. Focusing on key elements of each diagnosis will hopefully add to the clinician's efficiency and level of comfort in the evaluation and management process. The background section is followed by a discussion of assessment and, finally, treatment considerations. The particular approach to treatment will vary based upon the details of the case, clinician resources, and patient resources. Therefore, it would be short-sighted, and presumptuous, to outline a specific protocol. Unlike surgery or interventional therapy, this is primary care pain medicine. Treatment is longitudinal, and sometimes palliative, even in the noncancer chronic pain population. Key points are listed as a way summarizing each case discussion.

At the heart of it all is the assertion that chronic pain is a complex, dynamic, and a progressive disease process. In this sense, it is similar to diabetes and hypertension; there is no known cure. Left untreated, the problem often worsens. Genetics, environment, lifestyle, and incentives each play a role. It is incumbent upon the committed clinician, whatever his or her disciplinary training, to navigate this landscape and to piece together the best approach possible. The old adage of "Do not harm" applies. Some feel compelled to "do something"; be careful of that which cannot be reversed (e.g., surgery). The author has seen scores of patients improve as a result of natural consequences. At times, maintaining a presence through periodic office visit is sufficient.

Importantly, know your limits. We often speak of the psychology of the patient, but that of the clinician is equally relevant. Some clinicians can be very unassertive and even co-dependent. There is an apt saying relating to medication prescribing: "Don't say yes, if you can't say no." Some folks are very impatient with the patient; understandable. But try not to let treatment be about you instead of what is best for the patient.

There is a separate chapter on psychological/behavioral therapies following the section on case studies. This was done so that time would not be taken up explaining each technique during the case discussion. Some may want to read this section first to become familiar with the terms and techniques. Many of the psychological therapies can be quite involved. However, truncated and brief interventions can be useful and often are more practical. iPhone apps and the internet can be valuable resources. For those that do not have access to a pain-oriented psychological, telepsychology is on the horizon.

The lack for correlation between physical findings and the patient's complaints of pain, the continued emphasis on the multidisciplinary model, and the use of psychologically based therapies seem to support, if only at a subliminal level, chronic pain as a psychogenic problem. Some would see this as a straw-man debate, but the unfortunate manner in which some patients, especially those seen as refractory to existing treatments, are regarded suggests otherwise. The issue of psychogenic pain is addressed, and hopefully the reader will agree with the conclusion and its logic.

The chapter on the psychology of opioid tapering addresses some of the current issues surrounding the use opioids in managing the patient with chronic pain. The Centers for Disease Control and Prevention guideline of 2016 prompted the unleashing of a torrent of regulations and recommendations, which can be frightening to the patient and clinician alike (Dowell et al, 2016). The apparent pressure to taper and withdraw opioid medication appears to be driven more by psychological factors than scientific and clinical evidence.

The issues of medical marijuana, whatever this actually comes to represent, is, here to stay. Hemp and CBD (cannabidiol) products have become common place. However, product quality is highly variable and claims of benefit unsubstantiated. The clinician needs a basis of knowledge to communicate effectively with the patient and hopefully prevent harmful experimentation prompted by misleading advertising. Ironically, we find ourselves in a situation not to different from the 1980s when the use of opioids for chronic pain became acceptable. It is important to help patients discover self-directed therapies.

Often overlooked, if not ignored, are dietary supplements and nutrition. The amount of controlled research, including randomized controlled trials, is worthy of attention. The terms "alternative" and "complementary" are unfortunate, as many of these therapies should form the basis of other treatments. For example, research as to the role of inflammation has gained a good deal of attention. Many traditional medicines and therapies only address the consequences. There are variety of simple and cost-effective lifestyle changes that can yield meaningful clinical results. It can provide a response to the patient asking "What do I do now?"

Although not necessarily intended for this purpose, this book represents a useful study aid in preparation for board examination in the area of pain. The author has given many lectures for this purpose and has attempted to incorporated information that is concise and current.

Further Reading

Aydede M, Shriver A. Recently introduced definition of "nociplastic pain" by the International Association for the Study of Pain needs better formulation. *Pain*. 2018;159(6):1176–1177.

Dowell D, Haegerich TM, Chou R. CDC guideline for prescribing opioids for chronic pain—United States, 2016. *MMWR*. 2016;65(1):1–49.

The need of a taxonomy [Editorial]. *Pain*. 1979;6:247–252.

Quintner JL, Buchanan D, Cohen ML. Katz J, Williamson O. Pain medicine and its models: helping or hindering? *Pain Med*. 2008;9:824–834.

Case Studies

1   A Broken Life

Jack is a 48-year-old male with a history be being very active physically. As a result of a skiing accident, he has undergone three surgeries to his low back, including a multilevel fusion. He has chronic back and bilateral leg pain. Because of increased symptoms, he underwent updated testing and a surgical consult. Diagnostic testing reveals postoperative changes, degenerative changes at the disc level above the fusion, and arachnoiditis. He was told there was no surgical solution to his problem and that it would probably worsen as time goes on. His activity level is limited. He had to sell his small business. He has a wife and two children, one finishing high school and the other just starting college. Because of financial changes, they have had to sell the house they built and move to a smaller one. He has been cooperative with his treatment and is on a fair amount pain medicine but does not appear to responding as you would hope. Spinal blocks and modalities have been relatively ineffective. Although he does not acknowledge it, he seems very despondent and reports fatigue, insomnia, and some irritability.

What do you do now?

BACKGROUND

Depression is not a unitary concept. Its relationship to pain can be complex (Box 1.1). Studies have reported up to 85% of patients with chronic pain manifest symptom of depression. At times, depression may need to be addressed aggressively prior to other pain therapies; in other situations, it may improve along with pain reduction and improved function.

Pain can be a major risk factor for depression. In the presence of co-existing depression, patients with chronic pain have more pain complaints and report greater pain severity. In addition, they are up 4.6 times more likely to report functional impairment/interference with activities of daily living and to take sick leave because of pain than those having depression without pain. In the elderly, there is 9% chance of recovering if both diagnoses exist versus 47% if a single diagnosis. The cost of treatment is 25% to 50% higher and the patient's life span is shortened (Blair et al, 2003). In general, such patients are more recalcitrant to treatment and at higher risk for aberrant drug behavior. There is some evidence that neuroinflammation may be a common mechanism (Kaplan and Heimur, 2013; Doan et al, 2015).

The loss of self-esteem, one's identity, and sense of control combined with feeling hopeless is a breeding ground for depression. The patient, however, may experience this as part of his pain and not recognize it as depression, or they will view their pain and their life circumstances as the sources of the depression, believing that these must be resolved before the depression will improve. Jack's case is, unfortunately, not uncommon. Although

---

BOX 1.1 **Theories of Pain and Depression**

Antecedent: Depression precedes the development of chronic pain.

Consequence: Depression is a consequence of the chronic pain.

Scar: Episodes of depression occurring before the onset of chronic pain predispose the patient to a depressive episode after the onset of pain.

Cognitive mediation: Psychological factors (eg, poor coping) mediate the reciprocal interactions between chronic pain and depression.

Independent: Depression and chronic pain share some common pathogenetic mechanisms but remain distinct diseases without causal interaction.

not their fault, many in his situation feel guilty for what the family has to give up. In some cases, spouses have to go to work. College education has to be postponed or pursued only if scholarships or grants are available. The selling of possessions and downsizing can be embarrassing. Family and individual social lives are disrupted.

ASSESSMENT

Assessing for depression can take several forms: brief questionnaires, comprehensive testing (eg, Minnesota Multiphasic Personality Inventory), and psychological/psychiatric consultation. The acronym SIGECAPS (Box 1.2) represents a constellation of eight symptoms that can be easily elicited in a brief interview. In general, the presence of five or more every day for two weeks correlates highly with a diagnosis of depression. A positive response to asking the patient if in the last two weeks or more they have experienced persistent sadness and loss of pleasure or loss of interest in things also correlates nightly with depression. The Beck Depression Inventory and Patient Health Questionnaire are well-validated and take only minutes to administer and score. The latter is even available on a Smartphone app, allowing periodic home-based assessment.

Although the risk of suicide in relatively low, it is higher than in some other medical conditions. The incidence has recently increased secondary to some clinicians imposing ill-advised and inappropriate medication reduction in otherwise compliant and improved patients. This seems to have been

---

BOX 1.2   **SIGECAPS**

Sleep: insomnia or hypersomnia
  Interest: diminished interest and/or pleasure from activities (eg, previously enjoyable ones)
    Guilt: excessive or inappropriate guilt; feelings of worthlessness
    Energy: lack of or fatigue
    Concentration: difficulty concentrating, indecisiveness
    Appetite: increase, decrease, weight loss
    Psychomotor retardation (lethargy) or agitation
    Suicide: recurrent thought of death, suicidal ideation or attempt

prompted by an over- or misinterpretation of the 2016 Centers for Disease Control and Prevention guidelines, which were intended for the primary care physician (Dowell et al, 2016). Indeed, the guidelines recommend against involuntary aggressive reductions especially in well-established patients.

There is an element of grief that is not often unrecognized. It can take at least two forms. One is the loss of life that was, and the second, loss of a life that was to be. In the first instance, individuals grieve over the loss of income, independence, reinforcing activities, self-esteem, and pride. They tend to feel useless if they cannot function at the level they once did. Their identity is gone and life seems to lack meaning. In the second instance, the future that was to be—an active and a financially secure retirement, big weddings, and traveling with grandchildren—seems to have evaporated overnight. This grieving process can take three to five years to improve. Like other types of grief, some will resolve it faster than others. It responds better to individual therapy than just the use of medication.

TREATMENT

Even if you are uncomfortable treating depression in the context of chronic pain, a brief assessment can open the door for meaningful communication. Patients, especially men, resist this notion and fear they are being labeled as a "psych" case, and their pain, ignored. Helping the patient to appreciate depression as a common comorbidity and contributing factor to chronic pain early on and providing educational material can be effective.

The use of opioids can induce depression. An unintended consequence of opioid therapy is suppression of testosterone. The symptoms of hypogonadism (eg, moodiness, irritability, fatigue, insomnia, etc.) can mimic depression. A baseline medical evaluation, including routine labs, is always recommended before initiating chronic pain therapy. Assessing for hypogonadism should be part of this and should be updated annually for those on opioid therapy.

Antidepressant therapy, cognitive behavioral therapy, exercise, and supportive therapy have proven beneficial. Some patients will work their way through this on their own. What they need is an interested and sympathetic clinician willing to hang in there with them. All too often patients who do not respond immediately to a particular approach to their chronic pain are thought to be recalcitrant to treatment, informed by the clinician that there is nothing else to try, and referred on. If exposed to interventional therapy or neuromodulation before the depression is addressed, there is a significant change of a positive short-term response followed by a relapse. This only serves to magnify the feeling of helplessness and hopelessness that undergird depression.

There are several types of antidepressant medication tricyclic antidepressants, selective serotonin reuptake inhibitors, and the serotonin and norepinephrine reuptake inhibitors that have been approved by the U.S. Food and Drug Administration for the treatment of depression. Table 1.1 lists some of those that have been used to treat comorbid depression

TABLE 1.1. Some Antidepressant Medications Approved by the U.S. Food and Drug Administration for Depression That May Also Be Effective With Various Chronic Pain Conditions

Medication	Off-Label Use	Typical Dosing/Day (d)
Venlafaxine XR	Diabetic neuropathy	37.5–225 mg/d
Fluoxetine	Fibromyalgia	20–80 mg/d
Duloxetine	Diabetic neuropathy	60 mg/d (dosages >60 mg/d showed no benefit)
	Fibromyalgia	
	Chronic musculoskeletal pain	30–60 mg/d
		30–60 mg/d
Imipramine	Neuropathic pain	50–150 mg/d
Amitriptyline	Diabetic neuropathy	25–100 mg/d
	Chronic pain management	25–150 mg/d
	Migraine prophylaxis	10–150 mg/d
Nortriptyline	Chronic pain	10–150 mg/d
	Myofascial pain	12.5–35 mg/d
	Orofacial pain	10–100 mg/d
	Postherpetic neuralgia	10–160 mg/d
Desipramine	Neuropathic pain	25–150 mg/d

Sources: Williams AM, Knox ED. When to prescribe antidepressants to treat comorbid depression and pain disorders. *Curr Psychiat*. 2017;16(1):55–58, and Clark GT, Gutierrez MA, Venturin JS, Richeimer SH. Psychopharmacologic agents (antidepressants, antipsychotics, anxiolytics, and psychostimulants) used in chronic pain. *Pocket Dentistry*. Published January 5, 2015. Accessed November 1, 2019. https://pocketdentistry.com/8-psychopharmacologic-agents-antidepressants-antipsychotics-anxiolytics-and-psychostimulants-used-in-chronic-pain/

and pain. There are several mechanisms by which antidepressants can affect chronic pain. By virtue of their effect on serotonin, norepinephrine, and sodium channel blockade, antidepressants can modulate peripheral and central sensitization, as well as ascending and descending inhibitory mechanisms. The analgesic effect can be independent of their antidepressant action. They can impact insomnia, anxiety, and depression, making chronic pain more tolerable. Although an increased risk of suicidal thinking and behavior in children, adolescents, and young adults (aged <25 years) during the first two months of treatment have been reported, this has not been seen with adults over the age of 24. Indeed, a decrease risk of suicidality has been observed in those over the age of 65 years. These agents represent beneficial adjuncts to other therapies and a potential alternative to the use of benzodiazepines. As with nearly all medications, antidepressants are not without their side effects, the most common being dry mouth, constipation, urinary hesitation, drowsiness, blurred vision, postural hypotension, sweeting, and tachycardia.

KEY POINTS TO REMEMBER

- Chronic pain can be a life-changing event, and depression is common among patients with chronic pain.
- Many symptoms of depression can be effectively treated in the primary care setting.
- Having an affiliation with pain-oriented mental health practitioners can be an asset to you and your patients.
- Patients often develop a close relationship with their doctor. Becoming educated in basic assessment and treatment strategies relating to depression and chronic pain should be considered essential. Not all patients with depression require, or can afford, formal psychiatric/psychological intervention.

Further Reading

Bair MJ, Robinson RL, Katon W, Kroenke K. Depression and pain comorbidity: a literature review. *JAMA Intern Med*. 2003;163(20):2433–2445.
Doan L, Manders T, Wang J. Neuroplasticity underlying the comorbidity of pain and depression. *Neural Plast*. 2015;2015:504691. https://doi.org/10.1155/2015/504691

Dowell D, Haegerich TM, Chou R. CDC guideline for prescribing opioids for chronic pain—United States, 2016. *MMRW*. 2016;65(1):1–49.

Juurlink DN, Herrmann N, Szalai JP, Kopp A, Redelmeier DA. Medical illness and the risk of suicide. *Arch Intern Med*. 2004;164:1179–1184.

Kaplan G, Heimur J. Microglia: pointing us toward a new paradigm for understanding and treating chronic pain and depression? *Pain Practitioner*. 2013;23(4):27–32.

Haunted by Pain, Fatigue, and Insomnia

Tom is a 45-year-old male with a history of headache associated with neck and right shoulder pain following a motor vehicle accident three years ago. The headache appears to be muscular in nature. He has had an anterior cervical discectomy and fusion and arthroscopic surgery on his shoulder. He has pathology at the transitional cervical disc and degenerative joint disease in the shoulder. There is a fair amount of tightness in the right trapezius and occiput area. He has been through physical therapy and is reasonably compliant. Modality therapies are of some benefit. Despite your best efforts he complains of problems sleeping. He is currently taking a sedative-hypnotic and tranquilizer at bedtime. It seems clear that the lack of sleep is causing daytime fatigue, increased pain, and irritability. He also reports being "on edge" and easily startled.

What do you do now?

BACKGROUND

Posttraumatic stress disorder (PTSD) is characterized by exposure to a traumatic events. Box 2.1 lists the symptoms.

The symptoms and their impact can vary in severity: 30%, mild; 33%, moderate; and 36%, serious. The use of alcohol and/or drugs to facilitate emotional "numbing" and suicidal thoughts tend to occur among the serious type. A frequently overlooked aspect of PTSD is that it can emerge as a result of witnessing a traumatic event versus physically experiencing the event.

In some settings, such as Veterans Affairs hospitals, the problem is fairly common, affecting upward of 30% of veterans having served in war zones. In the primary care setting, patients, especially men, may be unfamiliar with the symptoms of PTSD and hesitant to admit having them, feeling they should be able to cope or that the symptoms will go away. About 3.6% adults had PTSD in the past year. The lifetime prevalence of PTSD was 6.8%. Past year prevalence was higher for females (5.2%) than males (1.8%; National Institute of Mental Health, 2017). The events are most commonly associated with the development of PTSD; the estimated percentage of individuals exposed to the event are list in Table 2.1.

Physical or sexual abuse is a common cause of PTSD. It is noteworthy that up to 48% of women referred to multidisciplinary pain reported history of abuse (Kendall-Tackett, 2008). One cross-sectional study of primary care clinics in Wisconsin found that 47% of women and 22% of men reported a history of lifetime physical abuse, and 35% of women and 10%

BOX 2.1 **Symptoms of PTSD**

- Intrusive thoughts, flashbacks and/or nightmares
- Psychophysiological reactivity (eg, pounding heart, rapid breathing, nausea) to cues of the event
- Avoidance/withdrawal, including selective amnesia, upon exposure to cues associated with or resembling those of the event
- Hyperarousal/vigilance, decreased sleep, increased startle reflex, loss of ability to concentrate
- Emotional changes (eg, emotional numbing, loss of interest, detachment, problems, irritability, anger, or rage)

TABLE 2.1 **Causes of PTSD by Percentage**

Event	Percentage
Natural disaster	14
Accident	19
Severe suffering	20
Weapon assault	32
Illness/injury	43
Transportation	40
Sudden death of loved one	43
Sexual assault/rape	57
Other sexual trauma	64
Physical assault	70

Adapted from Titov N, Solley K, Dear BF, et al, Characteristics and treatment preferences
of people with symptoms of posttraumatic stress disorder: an internet survey, *PLOS ONE*
2011;6(7):0021864.

of men reported lifetime sexual abuse among patients prescribed opioids for
chronic pain (Balousek et al, 2007).

PTSD can co-exist with chronic pain. It usually follows an amputation,
trauma, injury, or accident. If not identified and addressed, it can render
chronic pain more recalcitrant to treatment. Individuals with comorbid
pain and PTSD have more health problems, more pain-related disability,
higher pain ratings, and increased functional impairment.

Obviously, not everyone who is exposed to, or witnesses, a traumatic
event develops PTSD. Risk factors associated with its development of
PTSD are given in Table 2.2. The elderly are not immune to developing
PTSD. Several factors have been associated with the development of PTSD
in the elderly (Box 2.2).

ASSESSMENT

Lack of sleep can be contributing factor to many of Tom's symptoms including fatigue and increased pain. One should question about a possible

TABLE 2.2 **Risk and Preventative Factor Associated with the Development of PTSD**

Risk Factors	Preventative Factors
Previous traumatic experience	Strong support system
Family history of PTSD or depression	Obtained counseling
History of substance abuse	Felt good about one's actions during or response to the trauma,
History of physical or sexual abuse	Demonstrated effective coping strategies
History of depression, anxiety or other mental illness	Felt capable of acting and responding effectively despite fear.
High level of stress in everyday life	
Lack of support after the trauma	
Lack of coping skills	

sleep disorder, overuse of caffeine, and exercise. However, being on edge, easily startled, and irritable would also suggest the possibility of PTSD. Upon questioning about his sleep, Tom admits to difficulty falling asleep for fear of nightmares relating to the motor vehicle accident. During the day he overreacts to sudden loud sounds, especially of something breaking, like glass. Although he drives, he is overly cautious to the point of being

---

BOX 2.2 **Factors Associated With the Development of PTSD in the Elderly**

- Neurological illness/depression
- Grief over the loss of friends, family, or spouse, especially if suddenly
- Retirement coupled with more time to think about war
- Decreased physical condition
- Bad news of TV brings back memories
- Previous use of alcohol in one who no longer drinks.

---

disruptive to surrounding traffic. His headache seems worse when driving and in the morning.

It is now well established that specific areas of the brain are key to the development and maintenance of PTSD. These areas include the amygdala, hippocampus, and medial prefrontal cortex. The overactivity seen in some cortical structures may also be secondary to reduced regulatory efficiency in others. Hormones and neurotransmitters such as cortisol and noradrenaline appear to play major roles in PTSD (Bisson, 2009). Not surprisingly, there is a significant overlap between the brain structures and physiological mechanism involved in PTSD and the processing of chronic pain.

PTSD has been associated with dysregulation of the hypothalamus-pituitary-adrenal (HPA) axis and the hypothalamus-pituitary-thyroid axis. In general, PTSD patients have significantly lower plasma cortisol, prolactin, and thyroid-stimulating hormone (thyrotropin) levels. Furthermore, the severity of PTSD symptoms is negatively correlated with cortisol levels. In addition, the findings involving the HPA axis are different for PTSD than those usually associated with chronic stress. For example, (i) cortisol levels are lower in PTSD patients than in non-PTSD trauma survivors and normal controls, and (ii) circadian pattern of cortisol release is more dynamic in patients with PTSD than patients with major depression or in normal controls. Although frequently overlooked, the HPA also plays a significant role is certain types of pain, especially fibromyalgia.

From a psychological perspective, chronic pain and PTSD share two main features: fear and avoidance (Foa and Kozak, 1986). The perceived or real emotional/physical trauma set in motion the appearance of fear-based cognitions (catastrophizing; eg, "I could have died"; "What if he attacks again. How will I survive?"). These thoughts lead to hypervigilance and attempts to avoid the feared situation (avoidance behavior). To the extent that future trauma is avoided, this behavior is reinforced and strengthened. In extreme cases, the patient is all but behaviorally paralyzed. In short, the persistent avoidance of feared stimuli (pain- and trauma-related) is paradoxically considered to be adaptive. Although the pain persists, further damage and more severe pain is perceived to have been avoided. These continued thoughts and behaviors increase the perceived threat and negative salience of the individual's environment. It is easy to understand how some see their world as an accident ready to happen. Such strong beliefs and avoidance behavior are not likely to be resolved without psychological intervention. Merely treating the chronic pain, even if somewhat successful, rarely improves the PTSD symptoms.

The effects of PTSD (anxiety) can be indirectly propagated. For example, the offspring of mothers affected by the 9/11 attacks, have been shown to have a disproportionate predilection to the development of anxiety and stress related disorders. The study of epigenetics has suggested that although the DNA has not been altered, the genetic expression has. This is not unlike twin studies demonstrating the impact of environmental factors on genetic predispositions.

Evidence exist that suggests that traumatic events cause the formation of a cell assembly—a memory (aka fear networks; Lang, 1979). These cells can be encased by an extra-cellular matrix forming a type of perineuronal net (PNN). The presence of the PNN stabilizes established neuronal connections and restricts plasticity (reorganization) that would ordinarily occur within the central nervous system in response to new experiences. Disruption of PNNs can reactivate plasticity allowing activity-dependent changes to once again modify neuronal connections and thus existing memories (Wang and Fawcett, 2012; Chelini et al, 2018). Thus, prior to the forming of PNN, extinction can result in an unlearning and "erasure" of conditioned fear memories. However, in the presence of PNNs, "fear extinction *does not* erase previously acquired fear memories, but involves new learning eventually inhibiting conditioned fear behavior" (Emphasis added, Gogolla et al, 2009, p. 1258). Furthermore, encouraging the patient to ignore such memories initiates an ironic process (Wegner, 2009). Quite simply, it is what happens when one is told to "not think about pink elephants." There is an active nonconscious process that blocks certain thoughts/memories form consciousness (Dijksterhuis and Nordgren, 2006; Kihlstrom, 1987). Therefore, during distraction or suppression, intrusive memories are absent. However, there is the ironic rebound of suppressed thoughts when the person abandons efforts to suppress (eg, during sleep, revisiting the suppressed thoughts, or unusually intense mental load). Neurophysiologically, the presence of PNNs cause these cell assemblies (memories) to resist degradation and thus become recalcitrant to treatment.

TREATMENT

As always, treatment begins with the patient coming to understand the nature of their problem(s) and that their situation can improve. The presence of fear-avoidance cycles are involved with chronic pain and PTSD. These cycles are self-perpetuating and can spawn maladaptive beliefs, ineffective coping behaviors, distressing symptoms, and functional limitations. Treatment can be approached in several stages: (i) education emphasizing the importance of the interaction between behavior, emotion, and cognition (ascribing meaning or appraisals) to both chronic pain and PTSD; (ii) addressing avoidance behavior through structured situational exposure/confrontation exercises; (iii) treatment for depression; (iv) use of therapies (eg, cognitive restructuring, cognitive behavioral therapy) to challenge maladaptive thoughts and strengthen sense of self-esteem/efficacy; (v) correction of attentional biases that develop in response to both chronic pain and PTSD; and (vi) attempt to normalize emotional responses and contributing physiologic sensations (Bosco et al, 2013).

Table 2.3 lists psychological and pharmacological therapies that are proven to be beneficial in treating PTSD. Sertraline and paroxetine are both approved for use with PTSD. Prazosin has been successfully used to reduce nightmares, flashbacks, and sleep disorders.

Despite the complaints of anxiety, benzodiazepine drugs should not be a first-line therapy and ought to be used with great caution. Table 2.3 lists some reasonable options. Although not approved by the US Food and Drug Administration for use with chronic pain, antidepressants can influence serotonin and/or norepinephrine and may impact both PTSD and pain. In all likelihood, patients will require some behavioral/psychological intervention. If the notion of PNN holds, then desensitization to the emotional reaction associated with the memory and reduced startle reaction and avoidance behavior will need to be addressed. Most doctoral-level psychologists will have knowledge and experience in this area. The emergence of telepsychology and internet-based therapy may make treatments more accessible and the use of virtual reality technology, more efficient.

Opioids should be used with caution. The human body contains an endogenous opioid system capable of tempering a variety of psychological/psychiatric symptoms. The use of opioids may activate this system,

TABLE 2.3 **Treatment for PTSD**

Recommendations	Psychological Therapy	Psychopharamcology
First line treatment	Exposure therapy Cognitive behavioral therapy Eye movement desensitization and reprocessing	Sertraline Paroxetine Fluoxetine
Demonstrated benefit	Cognitive behavioral therapy–specific PTSD Narrative exposure therapy Brief eclectic psychotherapy	Venlafaxine Imipramine Prazosin
Some Benefit	Meditation-based therapy	Nefazodone
Recommend against		Monotherapy with antipsychotics, benzodiazepines, or medical marijuana

From Copra MP, PTSD in late life: special issues, *Psychiatric Times.* 2018;13(3). https://www.psychiatrictimes.com/ptsd/ptsd-late-life-special-issues. Accessed December 21, 2010.

suppressing some of the emotionally distressing feelings. The patient may feel some relief, but the problems is being masked. They may use opioids to calm distress rather than to improve function. Any attempt to reduce the opioids may be met with resistance for fear of symptom rebound. This can create a strong psychological dependence on the opioid (Sachy, 2010). However, there have been reports of opioid therapy for co-existing pain improving the PTSD symptoms. It is unclear if this reflects activation of the endogenous opioid system, a reflection of the relationship between pain and PTSD symptoms, or some combination of the two.

KEY POINTS TO REMEMBER

· The incidence of PTSD in patients with chronic pain, especially fibromyalgia and those associated with some type of trauma, is significant.

- One should inquire about PTSD symptoms and any history of trauma early on. Simply asking "At any point in your life as a child, adolescent, or adult have you ever been the victim and any type of abuse, assault, molestation, or abandonment. I do not need to know the details, only if it ever happened." The patient's expression itself may be very telling.
- Any patient presenting with chronic pain associated with some type of trauma/accident should be assumed to experience some level of PTSD until proven otherwise.
- Whenever possible, avoid the use of benzodiazepines and opioids.
- Maintain a list of psychological/mental health professionals to use a referral sources. Assure the patient that you are not abandoning them but obtaining some assistance to help address the complexity of their problem.

Further Reading

Balousek S, Plane MB, Fleming M. Prevalence of interpersonal abuse in primary care patients prescribed opioids for chronic pain. *J Gen Intern Med.* 2007;22(9):1268–1273.

Bisson JI. The neurobiology of post-traumatic stress disorder. *Psychiatry.* 2009;8(8):288–289.

Bosco MA, Gallinati JL, Clark ME. Conceptualizing and treating comorbid chronic pain and PTSD. *Pain Res Treat.* 2013;3:1–10. https://doi.org/10.1155/2013/174728

Cholini G, Pantazopoulos H, Durning P, Berrettaaet S. The tetrapartite synapse: a key concept in the pathophysiology of schizophrenia. *Eur Psychiatry.* 2018;50:60–69.

Dijkstorhuis A, Nordgren LF. A theory of unconscious thought. *Perspect Psychol Sci.* 2006;1(2):95–109.

Foa EB, Kozak MJ. Emotional processing of fear: exposure to corrective information. *Psychol Bull.* 1986;99:20–35.

Gogolla N, Caroni P, Lüthi A, Herry C. Perineuronal nets protect fear memories from erasure. *Science.* 2009;325:1258–1261.

Kendall-Tackett K. Chronic pain in adult survivors of childhood abuse. *Trauma Psychol Newsl.* 2008;Fall:20–24.

Kihlstrom JF. The cognitive unconscious. *Science.* 1987;237(4821):1445–1452.

Lang PJ. A bioinformational theory of emotional imagery. *Psychophysiology.* 1979;16(6):495–512.

National Institute of Mental Health. Post-traumatic stress disorder (PTSD). https://www.nimh.nih.gov/health/statistics/post-traumatic-stress-disorder-ptsd.shtml. Last updated November 2017. Accessed February 11, 2019.

Otis JD, Keane TM, Kerns RD. An examination of the relationship between chronic pain and post-traumatic stress disorder. *J Rehab Res Dev.* 2003;40(5):397–405.

Sachy TH. Use of opioids in pain patients with psychiatric disorders. *Pract Pain Manag.* 2010;10(7):17–26.

Vlaeyen JWS, Linton SJ. Fear-avoidance and its consequences in musculoskeletal pain: a state of the art. *Pain.* 2000;85:317–332.

Wang D, Fawcett J. The perineuronal net and the control of CNS plasticity. *Cell Tissue Res.* 2012;349(1):147–160.

Wegner DM. How to think, say, or do precisely the wost thing for any occasion. *Science.* 2009;325:48–50.

3 The Hand That Wouldn't Move

Devon is a 33-year-old female with a 10th-grade formal education, presenting with numbness involving the right (dominate) hand. It came on suddenly. She has some scares suggestive of minor injury to the hand. Although concerned, she also seems somewhat indifferent. She has not be able to work as a short-order cook. Absent insurance, she has not been able to seek medical help. The family reports that there has been some marital stresses and conflict, but nothing unusual. She has been somewhat sickly, but nothing serious. However, Devon has been acting somewhat peculiar as of late.

What do you do now?

BACKGROUND

Conversion disorder (CD), formally hysteria, was a common 19th-century diagnosis exclusive to women. Patients with a CD presented with blindness, deafness, pseudoseizures, dystonia, paralysis, syncope, or other neurological symptoms (Scott and Anson, 2009). The presenting symptoms depended on the cultural milieu and the patient's degree of medical knowledge. That is, the greater the degree of medical knowledge, the more subtle the symptom/deficit and the more closely it will simulate an actual medical/neurological condition; lesser knowledge is often associated with implausible symptoms. The symptoms can appear spontaneously and abruptly disappear. Duration is variable. CD is rarely threatening. But can be debilitating. It is estimated that about 5% of patients in a hospital setting, 30% of referrals to outpatient neurology clinics, and 24% of patients in psychiatric clinics meet the criteria for CD. These are mostly young adults. Women outnumber men up to 10:1. Some 48% of patients with CD also experience a dissociative disorder. Rates of CD are significantly higher in developed versus Third World countries. Box 3.1 give the diagnostic criteria and various symptom types from the fifth edition of the *Diagnostic and Statistical Manual of Mental*

BOX 3.1 **Conversion Disorder Diagnostic Criteria**

- One or more symptoms of altered voluntary motor or sensory function.
- Clinical findings provide evidence of incompatibility between the symptom and recognized neurological or medical conditions
- The symptom or deficit is not better explained by another medical or mental disorder.
- The symptom or deficit causes clinically significant distress or impairment in social, occupational or other important areas of functioning or warrants medical evaluation.

Source: American Psychiatry Association. *Diagnostic and Statistical Manual of Mental Disorders*. 5th ed. Washington, DC: American Psychiatry Association; 2013.

Disorders (American Psychiatry Association, 2013), and Box 3.2 lists symptom types.

There are three major theories relating to CD. The *psychodynamic* approach has its foundation in Freud. He believed the patient's anxiety was being "converted" into physical symptoms. Symptoms, therefore, have a symbolic relationship to an unconscious conflict (eg, vaginismus protects against the expression of unacceptable sexual wishes). The CD symptom is ignited by some psychological conflict or recent stressor resulting in an unconscious conflict between a forbidden wish (id) and the patient's conscience (superego). The conversion symptoms occurs without the patient's awareness of the unacceptable desire. The *learning* theory approach asserts that the symptom or symptoms are learned in childhood, through modeling or conditioning and emerge as a means of coping with an impossible situation. Finally, the *genetic* perspective hypothesizes that the conversion symptom is a result of dysfunctional cerebral hemispheric communication and excessive cortisol arousal that inhibit the individual's awareness of bodily sensations.

Functional imaging studies of the brain have revealed some interesting neurophysiological findings. One study (Marshall et al, 1997) examined woman with left-sided paralysis, without sensory loss or presence of an organic lesion. Attempts to move the paralyzed leg failed to activate the right primary cortex, as it should have. Instead, increased activity was seen in the right orbitofrontal and right anterior cingulate gyrus. The authors speculated that inhibitory pathways involving the orbitofrontal cortex and anterior cingulate may "disconnect" the premotor areas from the primary motor cortex, preventing the patient's conscious intention from being translated into action. Thus, it appears that inhibition of willed movement may play an important role in functional paralysis. It was further suggested that the presence of activation seen when preparing to move her affected limb provides evidence against feigning.

Vuilleumier et al (2001) argued that patients with a CD have a deficit in volition involving the left dorsolateral prefrontal cortex and striato-thalamo-cortical circuits. This explanation implicates different structures and functions then those previously discussed. It is possible, indeed probable, given the complexity of brain structure and function, that CD may be associated with deficits in both planning and execution (premotor stage). These data, however, do not reveal how or why these inhibitory or volitional pathways are activated.

ASSESSMENT

Diagnosing CD can be challenging. The symptoms generally do not conform to any anatomical pathway or physiological mechanism. A neurological examination including the hand-dropping test, saccadic eye movements, variable resistance, the Hoover test, unconscious movements, and the tremor entrainment test can help to identify symptoms that are inconsistent with true neurological pathology. A comprehensive psychological/psychiatric interview can help to uncover the onset of symptoms, temporally associated stressors, and psychological issues such as poor coping skills and internalized conflicts. CD may be comorbid with posttraumatic stress disorder, anxiety disorder, obsessive-compulsive disorder, etc. Table 3.1 lists a variety of risk factors that should be considered. A differential diagnosis involving factitious disorder, malingering, and somatoform disorder needs to be made. Psychological testing instruments such as the Minnesota Multiphasic Personality Inventory and neuropsychological tests can provided additional objective data and aid in differentiating CD from malingering.

The diagnosis of CD should be made after establishing positive clinical findings incompatible with organic disease. Table 3.2 lists some of the more

TABLE 3.1	Risk Factors for Conversion Disorder
Recent significant stress	Emotional trauma
Female vs. male	Late teens/early 20s
Rural population/lower socioeconomic status	Family history
Physical or sexual abuse/neglect	Mental health condition comorbidity
Neurological disease causing similar symptoms	Limited medical or psychological knowledge

common CD symptoms and how they differ from the condition they appear to be mimicking.

TREATMENT

Positive prognostic indicators in the treatment of CD include (i) sudden onset, (ii) short duration, (iii) early identifiable stressor, (iv) no ongoing litigation, (v) good premorbid functioning, and (vi) lack of comorbid psychiatric disorders. The key to successful treatment is the establishment of a strong therapeutic alliance and the incorporation of a goal-oriented treatment program. Many patients with CD are unable to understand the inner conflict, which is perhaps occurring on a nonconscious level. Confronting patients about the psychological nature of their symptoms can make the symptoms worse. However, patients can only achieve resolution of the conflict and the physical symptoms once they are able to recognize the connection.

Because patients tend to be less open to psychological explanations than patients with defined neurological illness, the groundwork for a discussion of psychological and stress-related factors must be approached carefully. Ali et al (2015) provide a number of recommendations (Box 3.3).

A variety of psychological therapies can, and probably should, be used with patients with CD. Individual/group therapy, behavioral therapy, hypnosis, biofeedback, and relaxation training can be useful. Cognitive-behavioral

TABLE 3.2 **Differentiating Features of Conversion Disorder**

Symptom	Features Differentiating CD Symptoms From Organic Disease
Psychogenic nonepileptic seizures	Patients generally lack response to treatment with antiepileptic drugs or have a paradoxical increase in seizures with antiepileptic drug treatment. A negative history of injury or loss of control of bladder or bowel during the seizure episode.
Tremor	When weights are added to the affected limb, patients with functional tremor tend to have greater tremor amplitude, whereas in those with organic tremor, the tremor amplitude tends to diminish.
Dystonia	Distinguishing features include an inverted foot or "clenched fist," adult onset, a fixed posture that is apparently present during sleep and the presence of severe pain.
Paralysis	The patient loses the use of half of their body or a single limb, but the paralysis does not follow anatomical patterns and is often inconsistent upon repeat examination.
Blindness	The patient complains of recent onset of blindness absent any injury or apparent cause. They do not display any expected bruises or scrapes. The pupillary reflex is present.
Syncope	The patient reports feeling faint or fainting, absent autonomic changes (eg, pallor). There is no associated injury. The fainting spells have a "swooning" character, heightening the drama of the event.
Anesthesia	May occur anywhere, but it is most common on the extremities (ie, the typical "glove and stocking" distribution). Unlike the "glove and stocking" distribution occurring in a polyneuropathy, the areas of conversion anesthesia have a very precise and sharp boundary, often located at a joint.

therapy has been particularly effective with pseudoseizures. Psychotherapy therapy should focus on (i) identifying the emotional bases of the symptoms, (ii) improving self-esteem, (iii) increasing the capacity to express emotions, and (iv) improving the ability to communication skills.

Physical and occupational therapy are necessary to prevent the potential long-term consequences of disuse. This is especially critical in the case where the CD symptom involve some level of paralyses. Therapy may be needed as long as the symptom persists. This also gives the patient a rationale for improvement. It is more acceptable for a symptom to improve as a result of physical versus psychological intervention. A graduated exercise protocol is usually best. While some aspect of therapy can be applied by the therapist (eg, modalities), it is necessary for the patient to be an active, rather than passive, participant.

CD can also be improved through the use of medications to treat underlying psychiatric issues, such as depression and anxiety. Medications may include antidepressants, anxiolytics, or others depending on the psychiatric comorbidity. Regular follow-up appointments with a neurologist and/or psychiatrist should be provided to the patient to limit emergency room visits and unnecessary diagnostic or invasive tests.

KEY POINTS TO REMEMBER

- Patients with CD are not malingering. Some providers falsely believe CD is not a real condition and tell the patient it is all "in their head."
- CD can cause distress and cannot be turned on and off at will.
- Symptoms usually begin suddenly after a stressful experience.
- Diagnosis is challenging and, to a degree, uses a "rule out alternatives" approach.

Further Reading

Ali S, Jabeen S, Pate RJ, et al. Conversion disorder—mind versus body: a review. *Innov Clin Neurosci.* 2015;12(5–6):27–33.

American Psychiatry Association. *Diagnostic and Statistical Manual of Mental Disorders.* 5th ed. Washington, DC: American Psychiatry Association; 2013.

Marshall J, Halligan P, Fink G, et al. The functional anatomy of hysterical paralysis. *Cognition.* 1997;64(1):B1–B8.

Scott R, Anson J. Neural correlates of motor conversion disorder. *Motor Control.* 2009;13:161–184.

Valleumier P, Chicherio C, Assal F, Schwartz S. Functional neuroanatomical correlates of hysterical sensorimotor loss. *Brain.* 2001;124(6):1077–1090.

4   Something Doesn't
       Seem Right

Rachael is a 38-year-old unemployed mother
of a teenager presenting for the first time with
complaints of neck, back, and gastrointestinal-
related pain. She reports a history of
unsuccessful treatments but has heard you are
a compassionate and carrying clinician. Subtle,
but well-healed scares are visible on her arms,
which she attributes to injuries during her active
youth. She is concerned that her current pain
medicine; although not effective, it will soon
run out causing severe withdrawal symptoms.
Her current clinician refuses to provide any
more. She seems very genuine, concerned, and
engaging. However, something just doesn't
seem right.

What do you do now?

BACKGROUND

It is necessary to differentiate between a personality *trait* and a personality *disorder*. Personality trait disturbance is an enduring pattern of perceiving, relating to, and thinking about the environment and oneself, exhibited in a wide range of social and personal contexts. A personality disorder is an enduring pattern of inner experience and behavior that deviates markedly from the expectations of the individual's culture; is pervasive and inflexible, with onset in adolescence or early adulthood and stable over time; and leads to distress or impairment. Personality trait disturbance does not meet the level of symptom severity and impairment as the personality disorder.

The fifth edition of the Diagnostic and Statistical Manual of Mental Disorders (American Psychiatric Association, 2013) describes borderline personality disorder (BPD) as a pervasive pattern of instability of interpersonal relationships, self-image, and affects associated marked impulsivity beginning by early adulthood and present in a variety of contexts. Box 4.1 list the features of the BPD.

The life-time prevalence of BPD ranges from 1.6% to 5.9%; about 6% in the primary care setting (American Psychiatric Association, 2013). BPD represents 15% to 25% of psychiatric illnesses; females out number males 3:1. BPD in males tends to be characterized by substance abuse and schizotypal, narcissistic, and antisocial personality disorders, whereas BPD in females tends to be characterized by posttraumatic stress disorder, eating disorder, or borderline identity disturbance. BPD is five times more common among first-degree biological relatives. The occurrence of BPD in people with chronic pain is about 30%, with a prevalence of up to 50% in the primary care outpatient setting, and is linked to increased pain severity and poor coping. Up to 80% of patients with BPD commit at least one nonsuicidal self-injurious (NSSI) behavior; cutting is the most prominent. However, 50% to 80% deny NSSI- associated pain, yet they report the act provides relief from aversive internal states.

NSSI is an auto-aggressive behavior patients use to decrease emotional pain and inner tension. It appears to do so by stimulating the release of the endogenous opioid and cannabinoid system, resulting in feelings of well-being, relaxation, and euphoria. Stress, often psychosocial in nature (eg, rejection) can result in a dissociative state and arousal of negative affect.

BOX 4.1 **Characteristics of BPD**

Five or more of the following are required:

- Frantic efforts to avoid real or imagined abandonment; may include suicide attempts or self-mutilating behavior
- A pattern of unstable and intense interpersonal relationship characterized by alternating between extremes of idealization and devaluation
- Identity disturbance: markedly and persistently unstable self-image or sense of self
- Impulsivity in at least two areas that are potentially self-damaging (eg, spending, sex, substance abuse, reckless driving, binge eating)
- Recurrent suicidal behavior, gestures, or threats, or self-mutilating behavior
- Affective instability due to a marked reactivity of mood (eg, intense episodic dysphoria, irritability, or anxiety usually lasting a few hours and only rarely more than a few days)
- Chronic feelings of emptiness
- Inappropriate, intense anger or difficulty controlling anger (eg, frequent displays of temper, constant anger, recurrent physical fights)
- Transient, stress-related paranoid ideation or severe dissociative symptoms

The rejection is often more perceived than real. NSSI tends to correlate with peak dissociative states. Patients with BPD often report the absence of physical pain, in combination with an increase in well-being/euphoria while engaging in NSSI. Thus, NSSI appears to have an antinociceptive function. These consequences tend to reinforce NSSI as a means of coping.

The likelihood of engaging in NSSI is associated with a history of suicidal thinking/behavior, unstable or inaccurate sense of self, recurrent impulsive behavior, and recurring/persistent feelings of meaninglessness. The tendency toward all-or-nothing thinking, intense and rapidly shifting emotions, and difficulties with emotional regulation can be exacerbated by distress, leading to maladaptive coping, which compromises both social and occupational functioning.

BPD has been the subject of rather extensive neurophysiological study (Ducassi et al, 2014). Structures that have been implicated included the anterior cingulate cortex, dorsolateral prefrontal cortex, insula, amygdala, and orbitofrontal cortex. Under- and overactivation of these cortical structures, when compared to normal, as well as altered connectivity, have been identified. Patients with BPD have an increased sensitivity to social rejection and decreased sensitivity to acute physical pain. Both physical and social pains tend to activate the pain matrix (including insula, cingulate, and secondary somatosensory cortices). In addition, research utilizing functional magnetic resonance imaging has discovered altered levels of gray matter density and activity in the anterior cingulate cortex and amygdala when compared to normal.

The complexity of the neuroanatomy and neurophysiology is reflected in this summary statement by Ducassi et al (2014):

> There are abnormalities in the affective–motivational and cognitive–evaluative pain components. Neuroanatomical studies have shown an exaggerated intracortical pain control associated with the reappraisal of stimuli, as well as attentional shift, decreased somatosensory attention, dysfunction of brain areas mediating the affective– motivational component of pain perception, and dysfunction in the central relay station, which integrates emotional and cognitive processes. Finally, SIB [self-injurious behaviors] (NSSI) may regulate psychological pain by increasing DLPFC, which is not activated enough through effortful psychological distancing, and by decreasing the activation of the amygdala. Repetitive SIB could attenuate pain sensitivity through repetitive stimulation of the endogenous opioid system. Finally, from the point of view of operant conditioning, SIB are negatively reinforced by reducing psychological pain. (p. 443)

Dysfunctions in serotoninergic, dopaminergic, and other neurotransmitter systems have been uncovered. Those with a history of repetitive NSSI had lower cerebrospinal fluid levels of beta-endorphin and met-enkephalin which are neuropeptides (proteins) associated with analgesia. NSSI may stimulate both the endogenous opioid system and dopaminergic reward system. The origin of these abnormalities could be severe childhood trauma, a biological predisposition, or some combination of these. Therefore, NSSI appears to prompt the body to release pain-relieving chemicals and induce a trance-like state that blunts physical and emotional pain. It is apparent that BPD has very complex neurobiological underpinning.

ASSESSMENT

As with many disorders, BPD symptom severity exists on a continuum. At one end are borderline traits consisting of emotionally immaturity, manipulation, and impulsivity; at the other end is the fully expressed disorder as reflected by seriously impaired social/occupational functioning, NSSI, and, at times, suicidality.

The patients with BPD frequently present announcing they have seen many other clinicians with little benefit. But, they have heard of you and are convinced you are the one who can help them. The young females with BPD can be very bright, clever, intelligent, and manipulative. They often are very alluring and disarming. They are the patient who may show up at your house or "accidentally" run into your spouse proclaiming how kind and generous you are. They frequently engage in splitting you and your staff. That is, they present to you as very gracious and cooperative, yet to your staff, they are defiant, augmentative, and demanding. This becomes apparent as your staff resists communication with the person you perceive as very accommodating. Remember Glenn Close's character, Alexandra "Alex" Forrest, opposite Michael Douglas, in the movie *Fatal Attraction*?

They will intentional or unintentionally misinterpret/understand what you have said. However, they are so convincing that you begin to doubt your own recollection. You may find yourself being talked into trying a therapy you find questionable. Thus, their manipulation can work, at least briefly. They are very apologetic for bothering you while you are on call, knowing how terribly busy you are and yet the calls continue. Therapeutic issues began to emerge, leaving you wishing you have never taken the patient on, but fearful of discontinuing treatment because of potential consequences hinted at by the patient.

One has to be weary up front. Learn to look for the signs. Outline the treatments and set the bar for continuation high. Never allow yourself to be alone with the patient—even if the patient insists o privacy to discuss a personal matter. Be careful of patients bearing gifts. Get records from previous clinicians. Do not short-cut the process. The patient with a BPD will be much more experienced at maneuvering and manipulating relationships than you. Listen to your staff. Insist on a psychological/psychiatric consult if you have any suspicion. Behavioral observations, appropriate history-taking, medical records, and searching the drug-monitoring data base are essential.

Patients with BPD with NSSI are different from those without co-occurrence of NNSI; likewise, differences exist between those who experience pain during NSSI and those who do not. Painful stimulation improves the dysphoric mood in BPD patients who do not perceive pain during SIB, but not in those who feel pain during SIB or controls. BPD patients without painful NSSI reported significantly reduced depression, anxiety, anger, and confusion subsequent to a provoked pain experience. Professing physical pain may provide a mechanism of gaining acceptance and care not otherwise achieved. However, the initiation of caregiving stimulates the patient's fear of rejection due to increased rejection sensitivity and a tendency to personalize others' intentions and emotional states. Because of this, they may begin testing the relationship. Patients with BPD show hyperarousal in response to negative emotional stimuli, leading to psychological pain. They have impaired control when experiencing social rejection and possess a dysfunctional empathic system that encourages sociopathic-like behavior.

TREATMENT

BPD predisposes individuals to a higher pain tolerance to acute (short duration) and self-inflicted pain, but lower pain tolerance, as well as greater pain severity and poorer coping, in response to chronic (ongoing) pain. Effective treatment and management of patients with BPD, especially those with NSSI, is beyond the scope and expertise of most primary care clinicians and pain clinicians; unless one is a trained psychiatrist. Specific treatments such as dialectical behavior therapy, schema-focused therapy, metallization-based therapy, and transference-focused psychotherapy have been developed. Dialectical behavior therapy has been shown to reduce NSSIB by up to 50% by teaching specific skills to reduce aversive inner tension and dissociation and the use of behavioral analyses to help the patient understand the antecedents and consequences of self-injury.

The patient, however, with chronic pain will most certainly request pain medication. They may accept less then requested as a means of 'establishing a doctor-patient relationship'. This empowers them to manipulate the situation. In any case, the use of an opioid or benzodiazepines should be avoided. Indeed, there are reports (Thürauf and Washeim, 2000) of the use of morphine-suppressing pain during NSSI but, paradoxically, intensifying the NSSI behavior. It has, therefore, been suggested that the use of strong analgesics might exacerbate BPD pathology. To the contrary, naltrexone, an opioid antagonist, appears to be helpful in controlling NSSI (Moghaddas et al, 2017). On the other hand, some patients with BPD and chronic pain may find that opioids alleviate other types of pain (eg, emotional pain or pain exacerbated by psychological distress), prompting drug-seeking or drug-overuse behavior.

Given the option, these patients may elect an office visit at the busiest time of the day or at the end of the day/week when you are most motivated to keep it short. Handle compliance issues yourself; do not avoid or deflect to your staff. Avoid getting caught up in a tug of war. This can be very reinforcing to the patient with BPD. Be prepared for a litany of reasons why most medications or therapies have not worked. They may not specify what they *really* want, except by excluding everything else. *Do not* succumb. One should neither ignore nor dismiss the patient's complaints of pain but insist upon a proper workup.

KEY POINTS TO REMEMBER

- Opioids in BPD with NSSI may enhance self-mutilation by suppressing the pain-induced stress-relieving effect of NSSI.
- BPD is a commonly encountered problem in primary care settings.
- The disorder is characterized by interpersonal problems, which often plays out in the relationship between doctor and patient.
- The underlying cause of the disorder is multifactorial and includes both brain abnormalities, genetics, and experiences early in life.

- The doctor–patient relationship can be greatly improved by better physician understanding of the disorder, good communication with all involved providers, minimization of polypharmacy, and learning how to respond to commonly encountered behavioral problems.

Further Reading

American Psychiatric Association. *Diagnostic and Statistical Manual of Mental Disorders*. 5th ed. Washington, DC: American Psychiatric Association; 2013.

Bandelow B, Falkia P, Schmal C, Wedekind DA. Borderline personality disorder: a dysregulation of the endogenous opioid system? Psychol Rev. 2010; 117(2):623–636.

Bohus M, Haaf B, Simms T, Schmahl C, Unckel C, Linehan M. Effectiveness of inpatient dialectical behavioral therapy for borderline personality disorder—a randomized controlled trial. *Behav Res. Ther.* 2004;42:487–499.

Ducasse, D, Courtet P, Olie, E. Physical and social pains in borderline disorder and neuroanatomical correlates: A systematic review. *Curr Psychiatr Rep.* 2014;16:443-455.

Linehan MM, Amstrong HE, Suarez A, Allmon D, Heard HL. Cognitive-behavioral treatment of chronically parasuicidal borderline patients. *Arch Gen Psychiatry.* 1991;48:1060–1064.

Magerl W, Burkart D, Fernandez A, Schmidt LG, Treede R. Persistent antinociception through repeated self-injury in patients with borderline personality disorder. *Pain.* 2012;153:575–584.

Minzenberg MJ, Fan J, New AS, Tang CY, Siever LJ. Frontolimbic structural changes in borderline personality disorder. *J Psychiatr Res.* 2008;42(9): 727–733.

Moghaddas A, Dianatkhah M, Ghaffari S, Ghaeli P. The potential role of naltrexone in borderline personality disorder. *Iran J Psychiatry.* 2017;12(2):142–146.

National Alliance on Mental Illness. Borderline personality disorder. http://www.nami.org/Learn-More/Mental-Health-Conditions/Borderline-Personality-Disorder. Reviewed December 2017. Accessed April, 2020.

Niedtfeld I, Schulze L, Kirsch P, Herpertz SC, Bohus M, Schmahl C. Affect regulation and pain in borderline personality disorder: a possible link to the understanding of self-injury. *Biol Psychiatry.* 2010;68:383–391.

Thürauf NJ, Washeim HA. The effects of exogenous analgesia in a patient with borderline personality disorder (BPD) and severe self-injurious behavior. *Eur J Pain.* 2000;4:107–109.

5   How Many More Are There?

Donna is a 39-year-old female seen on consultation while she is in the hospital. She has had three lumbar surgeries—the last, a multilevel fusion—and continues to complain of low back and leg pain. Her history is complicated by abuse in childhood, psychiatric treatment, and hospitalization. Despite information to the contrary in the medical record, she was very pleasant and forthcoming during the interview. She seemed fairly comfortable, and her mental status exam at the time was within normal limits. For the most part, her pain had been recalcitrant to blocks, pharmacological, and physical therapies. Options, including neuromodulation, are being considered. At the end of the interview she asks if you "want to speak to the others."

What do you do now?

BACKGROUND

Multiple personality disorder (MPD) came into prominence in 1973 with the publishing of *Sybil* and the subsequent film portraying the life of Shirley Mason. She was a psychiatric patient reportedly with 16 distinct personalities (alters), which she later admitted she faked. Nevertheless, this spawned an increase the frequency of MPD being diagnosed along with a flurry of research—both of which appear to have subsided.

The contemporary term for MPD is dissociative identity disorder (DID). The 12-month prevalence among American adults is estimated at 1.5%. Estimate of gender difference range up to 9:1, female over male. DID include elements of depersonalization, amnesia, derealization, and identity confusion/alteration. There are usually two or more personalities (identities, alters). Co-consciousness can occur. That is, the alters are aware and capable of using the body at the same time. Transitions from one identity to another are presumably initiated by psychosocial stress. However, at times, the patient appears to have some control over this transition. In the *possession form* of DID, the presence of an alter identity can be fairly obvious. In *nonpossession form*, one may not be immediately aware of any overt change.

The fifth edition of the Diagnostic and Statistical Manual of Mental Disorders (American Psychiatric Association, 2013) lists the diagnostic criteria for DID (Box 5.1). DID is usually associated with chronic and

---

BOX 5.1 **Diagnostic Criteria for Dissociative Identity Disorder**

- The individual experiences two or more distinct identities or personality states, each with its own enduring pattern of perceiving, relating to, and thinking about the environment and self (experience of possession or alters).
- The disruption in identity involves a change in sense of self and sense of agency and changes in behavior, consciousness, memory, perception, cognition, and motor function.
- Frequent gaps are found in the individual's memories of personal history, including people, places, and events, for both the distant and recent past.
- The symptoms cause clinically significant distress or impairment in social, occupational, or other important areas of functioning.

severe childhood trauma (eg, physical and sexual abuse, extreme and recurrent terror, repeated medical trauma, extreme neglect). The specifics of the etiology remain unclear, but the prevailing theory considers DID to be a reaction to childhood trauma. It is hypothesized that some severely traumatized individuals attempt to wall off, segregate, and dissociate the experience or memory via altered state of consciousness. Therefore, the victim mentalizes that the event happened to some other identity. Having a close relative with DID may be a risk factor, but a genetic link is yet to be established.

The validity of DID remains in question (Piper and Merskey, 2004a, 2004b). There are two dominant views. The nontrauma-related (NT; socicognitive) model asserts that "DID is a type of simulation associated with high suggestibility and/or fantasy proneness, suggestive psychotherapy, and other suggestive sociocultural influences (eg, the media and/or the church)" (Piper and Merskey, 2004a, p. 594). Whereas the trauma-related model (TR) views DID as a severe form of posttraumatic stress disorder emerging as a result of "chronic emotional neglect and emotional, physical, and/or sexual abuse from early childhood, insufficient integrative capacity, attachment disorder, and lack of affect-regulation by caretakers" (for a detailed discussion, see Reinders et al, 2012, p. 1). There appears to be a spectrum of responses to trauma (Box 5.2) ranging from acute distress disorder to DID.

The theory of structural dissociation of the personality (TSDP) asserts that there are many self-states—some are associated with trauma; others, with daily life. TSDP proposes the existence of two major prototypes of

---

BOX 5.2 **Posttraumatic Spectrum**

Acute stress disorder
Somatoform disorders
Simple posttraumatic stress disorder
Simple dissociative amnesia
Borderline personality disorder
Complex posttraumatic stress disorder
Dissociative disorder not otherwise specified
Dissociative identity disorder

---

dissociative parts (i) emotional parts (EP), and (ii) apparently normal parts (ANP). Defensive subsystems become rigid and fixated in traumatic experiences in the EPs. The ANP attempts to focus on daily life and activities while avoiding the traumatic memories and associated stimuli of the EP.

Neuroanatomical/physiological research, using positron emission tomography and functional magnetic resonance imaging technology, as well as psychophysiological measures, has demonstrated activation of different neural networks in DID patients versus controls and TR versus NT patients. TR patients tend to show activation in subcortical areas while NT patients show activation in areas of the cerebral cortex. This suggests that differential cortical processes are involved in modulating conscious and subconscious perception of trauma-related information. When listening to trauma-related descriptions, TR patients showed a shift in activation from the hippocampus to the caudate nucleus and amygdala—that is, a shift from brains areas associated with learning and memory to those involved in reflex-like flight-fright-freeze response. Interidentity amnesia (ie, not all of the alter personalities possess the same memories) exists, but the exact mechanism and causal circumstances are unclear.

DID involves dissociative part-dependent resting-state differences. Compared to ANP, EP-activated brain structures involved in self-referencing and sensorimotor actions are more active. Comparisons of neural activity for individuals with DID and non-DID–simulating controls suggests that the resting-state features of ANP and EP in DID are not due to imagination. The findings are consistent with TSDP and inconsistent with the idea that DID is caused by suggestion, fantasy proneness, and role playing.

There have been several reports of patients with chronic pain and DID/MDP. McFadden and Volker (1993) describe a patient with four different personalities, each reported different perceptions of pain. Psychological testing, visual analogue, the McGill Pain Questionnaire, pain drawing, and muscle activity as measured by electromyography were used. Each identity demonstrated a different pain perception, location, and estimate of secondary functional impairment.

The author has encountered five such patients over time. The majority were the possession form. One 45-year-old female failed to show for treatment during her four-week stay in a residential chronic pain program. She was found cowering, whimpering, speaking, and acting very much like a six-year-old child. She underwent two separate evaluations involving two different adult identities. Psychological testing and neurological and musculoskeletal data were different; the examiners were unaware of the two different alters. In four of the five cases, at least one of the personalities denied, and gave no indication of, being in pain. Furthermore, even though the personalities reporting pain used opioids regularly, there was no evidence of withdrawal syndrome when those who did not were present. On anecdotal and unpublished case report, the patient's psychiatrist reported a reduction of switching behavior when the patient's pain was controlled by the installation of a spinal cord stimulator. An increased was noted when the pain returned to baseline levels migration of the spinal cord stimulator electrodes.

Two reviews (Birnbaum and Thomann, 1996; Coons, 1998) have documented differences between personalities in physical symptoms, brain wave activity, visual-evoked potential, regional cerebral blood, visual function (eg, visual acuity, refraction, oculomotor status, visual field, color vision, corneal curvature, pupil size, and intraocular pressure visual refraction), muscle activity, cardiac and respiratory activity, galvanic skin response, dominant handedness, response to the same medication, allergic sensitivities, autonomic and endocrine function, and electroencephalogram.

ASSESSMENT

Several questionnaires have been developed for use in detecting DID. The Traumatic Experiences Checklist (Nijenhuis et al, 2002) is a self-report questionnaire assessing potentially traumatizing events such as physical abuse and emotional neglect. The Somatoform Dissociation Questionnaire (Nijenhuis et al, 1999) assesses the severity of somatoform dissociative symptoms (eg, analgesia, anesthesia, motor inhibitions). The Creative Experiences Questionnaire (Merckelbach et al, 2001) measures fantasy proneness.

In the clinic setting, DID of the possession type might be identified by remarkably different presentations. The appearance and demeanor of the different personalities may vary. History of trauma, marginal psychosocial adjustment/functioning, episodes of acting out/depression, periods of forgetfulness or memory lapses (ie, amnestic episodes), and history of psychological/psychiatric treatment may be clues. Simply asking if there are any "others" you need to talk with may be revealing. As always, it is the clinician–patient relationship that largely determines how forthcoming the patient will be. Questioning a significant other can also be informative.

TREATMENT

Psychotherapy is the mainstay of treatment. This may come in many forms including cognitive, family, and creative (art and music) therapies. Dialectical behavior therapy is a form of cognitive behavior therapy that aims to help the DID patient to decrease negative emotional and behavioral response to stressors using mindfulness-based therapy. Hypnosis may aide the patient in discovering information about their identity states and improving the level of control when transitioning from one state to another. Eye movement desensitization and reprocessing (EMDR) therapy facilitates the accessing of the traumatic memory network. Information processing is enhanced such that new and more adaptive associations can be created. Theoretically, these new associations result in complete information processing, new learning, elimination of emotional distress, and development of cognitive insights. In rare and extreme cases, electroconvulsive therapy can be a viable treatment when the combination of psychotherapy and medication does not result in adequate relief of symptoms.

Cure, in the sense of fully integrating the various identities into one personality, is unlikely. The goal of therapy is to achieve an adaptive coexistence of the person's multiple personalities. Patients are instructed in a ways to help identities to coexist and work together through developing crisis prevention techniques and coping strategies for dealing with lapses that occur during times of dissociation. This occurs by enhancing the communication between the various identities.

Guidelines for treating pain in DID patients are scant, if not nonexistent. Medications can be used to reduce levels of depression, severe anxiety, anger, and impulse-control problems that may contribute to the experience of pain. However, this should be left in the hands of a trained psychiatrist. Pain management should be done in conjunction with the mental health profession. Unfortunately, the DID patient with chronic pain may go undetected in a typical clinical setting. Vigilance should be heightened and suspicion aroused in the presence of highly inconsistent and erratic behavior, negative interactions with staff, and frequent issues of confusion or memory/forgetfulness. Although difficult to imagine, providing a certain type of medication, such as an opioid, to one personality, may be detrimental to another.

DID, unlike any other condition, leaves our understanding of pain as an open question. It is a remarkable experience to witness the transition from an identity with pain to one without and to engage in a meaningful interaction with both. The typical person who copes well with pain often speaks of dissociating themselves, via distraction or meditation, from it. Helping individuals develop these skills—even, if not especially, as children—could impact the development of chronic pain. Creating an overdependence on technologies, procedures, and medication may psychologically and physiologically compromise the development of these skills.

KEY POINTS TO REMEMBER

- There is strong evidence to support MPD/DID as a real phenomenon that is not entirely explained by fantasy proneness, motivated role-enactment, and suggestion.
- Physiological and neural activation patterns differ for DID patients versus normal controls.
- Treatment of DID should be deferred to experienced and trained mental health practitioners.
- The index of suspicion for DID should be raised in the presence of patients with erratic and/or inconsistent presentation, confusion, forgetfulness, social/occupation maladjustment, conflict with staff, and severe depression.
- "The problem is fragmentation of identity, not . . . that you have not more than one but less than one personality" (Spiegel, 2006, p. 567).

Further Reading

American Psychiatric Association. *Diagnostic and Statistical Manual of Mental Disorders.* 5th ed. Washington, DC: American Psychiatric Association; 2013.

Birnbaum MH, Thomann K. Visual function in multiple personality disorder. *J Am Optometric Assoc.* 1996; 67(6):327–334.

Coons PM. Psychophysiological aspect of MPD: a review. *Dissociation.* 1998; 1(1):47–53.

McFadden JI, Volker FW. Differing reports of pain perception by different personalities in a patient with chronic pain and multiple personality disorder. *Pain.* 1993;55(3):379–382.

Merckelbach H, Horselenberg R, Muris P. The Creative Experiences Questionnaire (CEQ): a brief self-report measure of fantasy proneness. *Pers Indiv Diff.* 2001;31:987–995.

Nijenhuis ERS, Van der Hart O, Kruger K. The psychometric characteristics of the Traumatic Experiences Checklist (TEC): first findings among psychiatric outpatients. *Clin Psychol Psychother.* 2002;9:200–210.

Nijenhuis ER, Spinhoven P, Van Dyck R, Van der Hart O, Vanderlinden J. The development and psychometric characteristics of the Somatoform Dissociation Questionnaire (SDQ-20). *J Nerv Ment Dis.* 1999;184:688–694.

Piper A, Merskey H. The persistence of folly: a critical examination of dissociative identity disorder. Part I. The excesses of an improbable concept. *Can J Psychiatry.* 2004a;49(9):592–600.

Piper A, Merskey H. The persistence of folly: critical examination of dissociative identity disorder. Part II. The defence and decline of multiple personality or dissociative identity disorder. *Can J Psychiatry.* 2004b;49(9):678–683.

Reinders AATS, Nijenhuis ERS, Quak J, et al. Psychobiological characteristics of dissociative identity disorder: a symptom provocation study. *Biol Psychiatry.* 2006;60:730–740.

Reinders ATS, Willemsen A, Vos H, den Boer JA, Nijenhuis ER. Fact or factitious? A psychobiological study of authentic and simulated dissociative identity states. *PLOS ONE.* 2012;7(6):e39279.

Reinders AATS, Nijenhuis ERS, Paans AMJ, Korf J, Willemsen ATM, den Boer JA. One brain, two selves. *Neuroimage.* 2003;20:2119–2125.

Schlumpf YR, Reinders AA, Nijenhuis ER, Luechinger R, van Osch M, Jancke L. Dissociative part-dependent resting-state activity in dissociative identity disorder: a controlled fMRI perfusion study. *PLOS ONE.* 2014;9(6):e98795. https://doi.org/10.1371/journal.pone.0098795

Spiegel D. Recognizing traumatic dissociation. *Am J Psychiatr.* 2006;163:566–568.

6 How Can Someone Do This to Themselves?

The only antidote for mental suffering is physical pain.
—Karl Marx

Charles is a 23-year-old male with history of alcohol and drug abuse, self-mutilation, a breaking and entering conviction, and suicide attempts. He was diagnosed with antisocial and borderline personality disorder. He inserted needles into his knees/ankles, pounded pieces of coat hanger wire into his abdomen and back, and swallowed open paper clips hoping they would become infected and kill him (see Figure 6.1). He had no complaints of pain.

What do you do now?

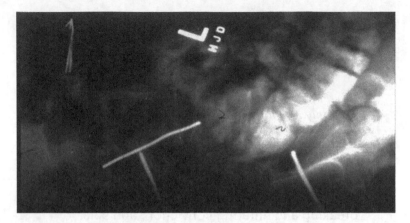

FIGURE 6.1 Example of self-injurious behavior.

BACKGROUND

Unless one is working in a hospital/psychiatric setting, you are not likely to encounter a case like the one previously described. Less dramatic forms may present at your office or emergency departments. Malingering (M) and factitious disorders (FD) did not appear in mainstream psychiatric classification schemas until the 20th century. They are considered abnormal healthcare-seeking behaviors, and some question considering the use of deception as a form of a mental disorder (Bass and Halligan, 2014; Bass and Wade, 2019). However, for our purposes, we will abide by the classification and interpretation of the fifth edition of the *Diagnostic and Statistical Manual of Mental Disorders* (DSM-5; American Psychiatric Association, 2013).

The essential feature of FD (Box 6.1) is the intentional falsification of medical or psychological signs and symptoms. There must be evidence of the patient taking covert actions to misrepresent, simulate, or cause signs or symptoms of illness or injury. This can include falsifying symptoms, events, and investigation results. Unlike M, there are no obvious external rewards. The underlining basis is often a psychiatric one (eg, the need to be a patient). The estimated prevalence is 0.5% to 2.0%.

Four subtypes of FD have been suggested. These include (i) a dramatic, deceptive, hostile, sociopathic wandering type, mostly male (Munchausen's syndrome), about 10% of cases; (ii) self-induced infections, mainly chronic or acute on chronic, largely female; (iii) willful interference with chronic wounds and cutaneous ulcers; and (iv) the simulation of disorders by falsification of data and fabrication of signs, symptoms, and physiological disturbances.

M is not considered as a mental disorder (Box 6.2). It refers to one who consciously and with malice of forethought, if you will, fabricates or significantly embellishes physical or psychological symptoms. M is motivated by an external reward, (eg, avoiding military duty, avoiding work, obtaining financial compensation, evading criminal prosecution, obtaining drugs). Many do not recognize that it is a federal offense (prescription fraud) to misrepresent one's condition for the purpose of obtaining a controlled substance; punishable by a jail sentence, fine, and loss of driver's license for six months.

The DSM-5 states that M is the only condition where symptoms appear solely because of an external incentive; differentiating it from FD, conversion disorder, and somatic symptom disorder. According to DSM-5, if any combination of the four items in Box 6.2 is present, you should consider the condition of M.

The incidence of M varies across diagnoses (Table 6.1).

As regards chronic pain, in particular, Aronoff et al (2004) reviewed several papers and found that the incidence of M ranges from 1.25% to 20%,

TABLE 6.1   **Incidence of Malingering by Diagnosis**

Diagnosis	Incidence (%)
Personal injury	29
Disability	30
Medical	8
Criminal	19
Chronic pain	31
Electrical injury	22
Fibromyalgia/chronic fatigue	35
Mild traumatic brain injury	39
Moderate to severe traumatic brain injury	9%
Neurotoxic Exposure	26%

From: Mittenberg W, Patton C, Canyock, Condit DC, Base rates of malingering and symptom exaggeration, *J Clinical Experi Neuropsychology,* 2002;24:1094–1102.

compared to 5% to 50% feigned mental disorders, and 7.4% to 67% for feigned cognitive impairment.

Several types of M have been proposed. The *pathogenic model* is characterized by a severe underlying psychopathology. The *criminological model* is made up of antisocial, noncompliant, and personality disordered patients. Finally, *adaptational model* consists of individual attempting to cope with adverse circumstances. The latter could be exemplified by a destitute person exaggerating symptoms or threatening suicide to gain refuge from the elements in the hospital, if only for a day or two. At least he would get dry clothes, a warm bed, and hot meals compared to eating a soggy, half-eaten sandwich extract from a trash can, and sleeping huddled against a cold brick wall with cardboard as the only cover.

ASSESSMENT

The assessment of both FD and M is much like detective work. Common to both FD and M is a detailed interview that seeks to determine the patient's motivations and level of conscious awareness regarding their reported symptoms. In the case of FD, a detailed examination of medical records is likely to reveal a very complex history including an unexpectedly large number of childhood illnesses and operations, high rates of substance abuse, mood disorder, and personality disorder. *Electronic FD* describes those who falsify their electronic medical records by creating factitious reports such as cancer.

When possible, medical records should be reviewed in advance of seeing the patient and guide the interview by inquiring about inconsistencies and specific events. General practice notes can be instrumental in proving a longitudinal perspective of the chronology of symptoms, treatments, and outcomes. This may require the efforts of more than one clinician. FD and M patients often count on the clinician being too busy to collect and review their records. Privacy and confidentiality regulations may compromise one's ability to secure medical records. Refusal to sign a release for records should create suspicion.

The FD usually has a history of multiple doctors and hospitals and using a fake name. The diagnosis of FD should be based on objectively identifying symptoms that are "manufactured" versus the patient's intent or motivation for doing so. A clinician should suspect FD when a review of the patient's history warrants it (Box 6.3).

BOX 6.3 **What to Search for in the Patient's History**

- The person's medical history doesn't make sense.
- No believable reason exists for an illness or injury.
- The illness does not follow the usual course.
- There is a lack of healing for no apparent reason, despite appropriate treatment.
- There are contradictory or inconsistent symptoms or lab test results.
- The person resists getting information from medical records, health care professionals or family members.
- The person is caught in the act of lying or causing an injury.

Most FD patients are likely to be socially conforming young women with stable social networks who present to general hospitals in their mid-30s. In the case of women, the self-induced illnesses begin in adolescence. Up to 50% these patients work in health-related occupations. Many patients have had childhood adversity and have coexisting chronic and complex somatoform disorders.

Most research on M takes place within specific legal contexts or when a patient attempts to evade punishment in the criminal justice system, seek damages through personal injury litigation, or gain financial compensation, whereas FDs are generally encountered in clinical settings. Aspects of the assessment are in Box 6.4.

Detecting the patient that is M is not always easy. Studies in this area make use of a standardized (lying) patient. These experimental confederates are well trained, rehearsed, and coached. In general, studies suggested that standardized patients were detected, or suspected, between 9% to 18%

BOX 6.4 **Aspects of the Assessment of Malingering**

- Review of medical records
- History obtained by interviewing
- Observation of the patient's behavior during the assessment
- Formal psychological/neuropsychological testing
- Symptom validity testing (if available),
- Surveillance video, when available

of the time (Jung and Reidenberg, 2007). However, don't be discouraged, even psychologists/ psychiatrists are little better at detection than other professionals or the lay public (Drob et al, 2009). Most healthcare professionals are not trained to determine the extent of a patient's (i) conscious awareness of the inconsistencies, (ii) conscious intent to deceive others, and (iii) the nature of any intention to deceive.

TREATMENT

In a litigiously oriented society, the clinician is all but compelled to give the patient the benefit of the doubt. Once medical investigation and/ or treatment is instigated, the patient can become relentless at insisting that it persist. The clinician would do well to fortify their suspicions and actions by obtaining a second opinion and/or psychiatric/psychological consultation. The initial diagnosis of FD, especially in a hospital setting, is most often made by a nonpsychiatrist. Most clinicians are ill-equipped to deal with the problem and should consult a psychiatrist. Recovery from FD is extremely rare, and very few patients agree to comply with treatment.

The treatment of the FD and M differ significantly. Management of the FD patient can be divided into two phases: acute and chronic. Acute management may well be carried out carried in an inpatient settings, emergency room, or an inpatient infectious diseases unit. Chronic management involves a long-term process of engaging the patient in some form of psychotherapy and harm reduction intervention. Many FD patients will manifest severe psychopathology or borderline personality disorder. The key to successful management in both phases requires negotiation and agreement of the diagnosis with the patient and engagement of that patient with treatment (Box 6.5).

Supportive confrontation if often required. It is best to involve at least two clinicians. The emphasis needs to be on helping the patient to realize they are in need of help. Management of the condition rather than cure is the focus of treatment. Treatment usually involve several components.

Hopefully, at a minimum, additional invasive or risky treatments can be avoided. In cases where the FD is imposed on others, the appropriate authorities may need to be involved.

Treatment of the M patient is somewhat different as one is not as likely to be dealing with a severe underlying psychiatric disturbance. A key question is, Does the M patient have the capacity to change their behavior? Perhaps the most common treatment involves a group feedback model involving (i) establishing rapport with the patient, (ii) exploring reasons for poor effort and /or acknowledgment of possible task disengagement, (iii) outlining the reasons for exaggeration, and (iv) discussing factors that can underlie symptom persistence. The data suggest that following confrontation as many as 67% of patients thought to have malingered tests performed in a nonforensic setting produced valid scores upon re-examination.

KEY POINTS TO REMEMBER

· FD is very complex and often involves serious psychiatric issues. One should not try to tackle these patients alone.
· Patients who malinger are not always easy to detect. They count on the clinician not having or taking time to investigate their situation fully.
· Have appropriate guidelines and procedures involving the prescribing of controlled substances in place; follow them.
· Patients who are malingering like to arrange appointments at the busiest and most inconvenient times.

Further Reading

American Psychiatric Association. *Diagnostic and Statistical Manual of Mental Disorders*. 5th ed. Washington, DC: American Psychiatric Association; 2013.

Aronoff GM, Mandel S, Genovese E, Maitz EA, Dorto AJ, Klimek EH, Staats TE. Evaluating malingering in contested injury or illness. *Pain Practice*. 2007;7(2):178–204.

Bass C, Halligan P. Factitious disorders and malingering: challenges for clinical assessment and management. Lancet 2014;383:1422–1432.

Bass C, Wade DT. Malingering and factitious disorder. *Pract Neurol*. 2019;19(2):96–105. https://doi.org/10.1136/practneurol-2018-001950

Drob SL, Meehan KB, Waxman SE. Clinical and conceptual problems in the attribution of malingering in forensic evaluations. *J Am Acad Psychiatry Law*. 2009;37:98–106.

Feldman M, Yates G. *Dying to be ill*. New York, NY: Routledge, 2018.

Folks, D. Munchausen syndrome and other factitious disorders. *Neruolog Clin N Am*. 1995;13:267–281.

Greve KW, Ord JS, Bianchini KJ, Curtis KL. Prevalence of malingering in patients with chronic pain referred for psychologic evaluation in a medico-legal context. *Arch Phys Medic Rehab*. 2009;90 (7):1117–1126.

Jung B, Reidenberg MM. Physicians being deceived. *Pain Med*. 2007;8:433–437.

Mittenberg W, Patton C, Canyock, Condit DC. Base rates of malingering and symptom exaggeration. *J Clinical Experi Neuropsychology*. 2002;24:1094–1102.

Turner J, Reid S. Munchausen's syndrome. *Lancet*. 2002;359 (9303):346–349.

7   An All-Consuming Problem

Jason is a 25-year-old male referred by a local
pain anesthesiologist. He is casually dressed,
appropriately groomed, and generally pleasant
in his manner. He is complaining of uncontrolled
low-back pain and compromised function.
A recent magnetic resonance image indicated
multilevel spondylitic changes with some
stenosis. A review of the prescription drug
monitoring program indicates he has been on
Suboxone® for 1.5 years with no indication of
"doctor shopping." He was informed early in
the interview that his use of Suboxone® would
potentially affect what would be prescribed.
When asked about the basis for using
Suboxone®, he readily admitted to a history of
heroin use, the most recent being one-year ago.
Further questioning revealed a five-year history
of being a "street addict" and HIV positive. When
heroin was not available, he used whatever he
could get. He entered a community-based clinic
and is being treated with Suboxone®, which he
had recently withdrawn himself from. He also
acknowledged daily marijuana use. He does not
want methadone or any other opioid associated
with significant withdrawal syndrome.

What do you do now?

BACKGROUND

It is important to clarify the terminology when discussing this topic as there tends to be a good deal of misunderstanding (Box 7.1).

The incidence of addiction in the chronic pain population has been estimated at about 2% to 5%. Some 20% will abuse their medication and about 40% will have one or more episodes of misuse (Webster and Webster, 2005). However, Barry et al (2010) reported that up 24% of chronic pain patients to be addicted or currently abusing opioids. Estimates of opioid use disorders (OUDs) in the primary care setting range up to 32%. Although lower, the incidence among those with cancer-related pain is about 7%. In their review article, Chang and Compton (2009) noted that 3.3% to

---

BOX 7.1 **Terminology**

Misuse: Use of a medication prescribed for a medical purpose other than as directed or as indicated, whether willful or unintentional, and whether harm results or not.

Abuse: Any use of an illegal drug. The intentional self-administration of a medication for nonmedical purpose (eg, altering one's state of consciousness).

Diversion: The intentional removal of a medication from legitimate and dispensing channels.

Addiction: A primary, chronic, neurobiological disease, with genetic, psychosocial, and environmental factors influencing its development and manifestations. Behavioral characteristics include: impaired control over drug use, compulsive use, continued use despite harm, craving.

Pseudoaddiciton: Syndrome of abnormal behavior resulting from under-treatment of pain misidentified as inappropriate drug-seeking behavior. Behavior ceases when adequate pain relief is provided. Not a diagnosis; rather, a description of the clinical intention.

Physical dependence: state of adaptation manifested by a drug class specific withdrawal syndrome produced by abrupt cessation, rapid dose reduction, decreasing blood level of the drug, and/or administration of an antagonist.

Tolerance: a state of adaptation in which exposure to a drug induces changes that result in a diminution of one or more of the drug's effects over time.

Based on Katz, NP, Adams, EH. Benneyan, JC, Foundations of opioid risk management, *Clin J Pain*. 2007;23(2):103–118.

11.5% of patients with chronic pain and a history of substance use disorder (SUD) develop opioid addiction or abuse, compared to 0.19% to 0.59% of those without a prior or current history of SUD.

ASSESSMENT

The fifth edition of the *Diagnostic and Statistical Manual of Mental Disorders* (American Psychiatric Association, 2013) uses the term "substance use disorder" to replace "substance abuse" and "substance dependence." SUD can be classified as mild, moderate, or severe based on the number of criteria met (see Box 7.2). When the substance involved is an opioid, the term "opioid use disorder" is preferred. SUD is appropriate when the recurrent use of alcohol and/or drugs causes clinically and functionally significant impairment; failure to meet major responsibilities at work, school, or home; impaired control; and risky use. Severe SUD is usually considered as synonymous with addiction.

It is important to understand the nature of SUD/OUD and addiction. There is the unfortunate tendency to equate the presence of tolerance and withdrawal with addiction. Opioid-induced hyperalgesia (Eisenberg et al, 2015) can also be confused with tolerance or even SUD. A key difference is that pharmacological tolerance can be overcome by increasing the dose whereas in the case of opioid-induced hyperalgesia, this will exacerbate the pain. Furthermore, patients demonstrating any kind of aberrant drug behavior (eg, self-adjusting the dosage, misplacing medicine, or requesting an early refill) are often inappropriately labeled as "drug addicts." Once this label becomes part of the medical record, it can significantly bias others against the patient, when, in fact, there may be other reasons for the behavior.

Although related, there is a difference between OUD and Addiction. As noted in Box 7.1, the American Society for Addiction Medicine (2019) defines addiction as

> a primary, chronic disease of brain reward, motivation, memory and related circuitry. Dysfunction in these circuits leads to characteristic biological, psychological, social and spiritual manifestations. This is reflected in an individual pathologically pursuing reward and/or relief

BOX 7.2 **Substance Use Disorder: DSM-5 Criteria**

Impulse control

- Use in larger amounts or longer than intended
- Desire or unsuccessful effort to cut down
- Great deal of time using or recovering
- Craving or strong urge to use

Social impairment

- Role obligation failure
- Continued use despite social/interpersonal problems
- Sacrificing activities to use or because of use

Risky use

- Use in situations where it is hazardous
- Continued use despite knowledge of having physical or psychological problem caused or exacerbated by use

Pharmacology[a]

- Tolerance
- Withdrawal

The severity of substance use disorder is based on

- 0–1 criteria: no diagnosis.
- 2–3 criteria: mild substance use disorder.
- 4–5 criteria: moderate substance use disorder.
- 6 or more criteria: severe substance use disorder.

[a]Although tolerance and physical withdrawal symptoms are listed among the 11 criteria, the fifth edition of the *Diagnostic and Statistical Manual of Mental Disorders* (American Psychiatric Association, 2013) explicitly states these are *not applicable* if the individual is under appropriate medical supervision.

by substance use and other behaviors. Addiction is characterized by inability to consistently abstain, impairment in behavioral control, persistent craving, diminished recognition of significant problems with one's behaviors and interpersonal relationships, and a dysfunctional emotional response. Like other chronic diseases, addiction often involves cycles of relapse and remission. Without treatment or engagement in recovery activities, addiction is progressive and can result in disability or premature death.

Addiction is often characterized by the five *C*s: chronic, compulsive, craving, loss of control, and continued use despite harm. Addiction should be confused with tolerance or withdrawal syndrome. The term "addiction" has been used interchangeably with severe OUD.

The case of Jason illustrates several points regarding assessment. First, when possible, one should have a screening process in place including obtaining records from previous treatment. Ideally, these should be reviewed before seeing the patient. In this case, the referring clinician did not carry out a detailed history prior to performing an ineffective block. The prescription drug monitoring program data did create some suspicion about the patient's history. Ordinarily, Suboxone® is prescribed for SUD ("Suboxone," n.d.). This patient displays a pattern consistent with addiction and should be treated in a specialized fashion. Second, a brief screening interview can save time by identifying and triaging patients to the appropriate resource. Third, patients will often use the presence of abnormal radiological finding as supportive evidence for the need of opioid therapy. The lack of correlation between physical finding and pain/function is well documented.

After obtaining information regarding his drug use history, including that the patient was not participating in a recovery program, he was politely informed that he would be a possible candidate for physical therapy, pain-psychological intervention, and the use of nonopioid agents. There are variety of nonopioid preparation that have been shown to have some analgesic properties. Preparations with a high potential for abuse (ie, benzodiazepines) should be avoided. When offered this course of treatment, the patient declined.

TREATMENT

There are some, but very limited, data on the use of opioids for the treatment of chronic pain in the addicted population (Dunbar and Katz, 1996). In this study, patients actively involved in a recovery program fared substantially better than those not involved. Patients in this category, or those determined to have a moderate or severe SUD, must be considered at high risk for aberrant drug behavior, and their treatment adjusted accordingly. This may require more frequent office visits, pill counts, drug screens, etc. This can be time consuming and is best carried out be a multidisciplinary clinic with adequate resources. A prime objective of the prescribing clinician is to prevent diversion. Addicts are likely to sell their prescribed opioid to obtain a stronger illicit drug. Although frequently overlooked because of the potential severity of their condition, diversion of this type can occur in the cancer pain population as well.

Successful pain management involving the patient in recovery or determined to be addicted in the primary care setting can be daunting. Some of the challenges facing the clinician are (i) distinguishing between seeking pain relief and seeking drugs for the euphoric effects, (ii) identifying predictable neuroadaptations such as tolerance and physiologic dependence that can be misinterpreted as drug seeking or relapse behavior, and (iii) comorbid psychiatric and medical conditions that can complicate treatment.

The use of controlled substances, especially opioids, may well be contraindicated. The presence of tolerance may mitigate against the effectiveness of these drugs. In addition, for those who are undergoing rehabilitation, opiate medications may trigger a relapse into their addiction. Furthermore, the Drug Enforcement Administration has expressed concern about the appropriateness of prescribing opioids to a patient with a history of addiction or or drug abuse, especially in the presence of a positive urine drug test for an illicit drug. Doing so, may contribute to diversion as it provides the patient with the opportunity to sell the proscribed medication as a means to obtain their drug of choice.

If treatment, especially with opioids, is considered appropriate, it should be consistent with established and accepted guidelines such as those of the American Academy of Pain Medicine (n.d.), and the Federation of State Medical Boards (2017). Individual state medical boards are likely to have their own guidelines. Prater et al (2002) provide some basic principles and case illustrations. They highlighted the importance of recognition and attention to concerns over withdrawal, relapse triggers, comorbid conditions, and proactive support for long-term recovery.

Emphasis should be placed on functional improvement versus pain reduction and use of a functionally oriented physical therapist. Co-management with a pain psychologist can minimize the feeling that one is going it alone. Compliance with recommendations to engage in these types of therapy can be a condition for initiating and maintaining medically based treatment.

There has been heightened emphasis on recognizing the disease aspect of addiction and providing appropriate services to the addicted patient in the midst of the opioid crisis, including medication assisted treatments (MATs; Volkow et al, 2014). MATs involve the use of methadone, buprenorphine, or naltrexone. MAT medications for OUD/SUD, which can only be dispensed through a clinician certified by the Substance Abuse and Mental Health Service Administration. This requires some additional training, which can be obtained online. The MAT should include counseling and behavioral therapies.

Suboxone' (buprenorphine hydrochloride and naloxone hydrochloride), for example, under the Drug Addiction Treatment Act (codified at 21 U.S.C. 823) is approved for use in the treatment of opioid dependence and limited to use by qualified physicians. The intent to treat opioid dependence and the assigned unique identification number must be included on every prescription. MAT is *not* simply substituting one drug for another. Rather, these agents are designed to relieve the withdrawal symptoms and psychological cravings. MAT agents help to suppress these symptoms and cravings, which can cause chemical imbalances in the body. They have no adverse effects on mental capability, physical functioning, or employability and, at the proper dose, can be taken safely for an extended period of time. They are most effective when used in combination with some type of recovery program.

The use of methadone in the treatment of addiction is restricted to licensed methadone treatment programs. It is illegal to write a prescription for methadone for the treatment of an OUD. Furthermore, any patient previously treated in a methadone program is considered to have an addiction/abuse diagnosis, limiting what can be prescribed in a pain management setting. Methadone is a full opioid agonist, while buprenorphine is a partial opioid agonist with a ceiling effect and therefore is much less likely to cause severe respiratory depression or overdose. Furthermore, methadone has been associated with increased pain sensitivity, thus complicating treatment (Compton et al, 2000). The patient with a poorly controlled mental illness, polysubstance use, and a chaotic environment may be better served in a methadone maintenance program wherein they are monitored daily (Beauchamp et al, 2014).

In the case of Jason, the most expedient action would be to assertively inform the patient you have nothing to offer, escort him out of the clinic, and suggest he not return. However, there is another more compassionate tactic to consider. Although not a candidate to be treated in your office/clinic you may be able to help Jason. The presence of hypogonadism as common among addicts is well established (Azizi et al, 1973). Hypogonadism can affect sleep pain, energy, mood, and bone demineralization (Kumar et al, 2010). Suggesting he get this checked and offering to make a referral to a recovery program would indicate that you are not summarily dismissing him because of his addiction. Also, informing the patient of the availability of Narcan*—in many states, offered over the counter—could save a life.

Psychologically speaking, good communication skills can influence the outcome. Even if the patient rejects all recommendations, clinicians can feel satisfied with their efforts. You never know when it will take hold. The author was surprisingly, and spontaneously, presented with a former patient's three-year abstinence pin as a result of the direct communication with the patient and wife when he was discovered years before to be using cocaine while in treatment for his chronic pain.

KEY POINTS TO REMEMBER

- A careful screening can be valuable to the clinician and patient.
- Understand the difference between abnormal drug behavior, SUD/OUD, and addiction.
- Do not try to treat problems beyond your level of comfort, training, and experience or the capacity of your office/clinic.
- Use the resources available to you such as comprehensive pain clinics and addiction recovery clinics.
- Above all, remember that effective, compassionate, and direct communication is always the best strategy.

Further Reading

American Academy of Pain Medicine. AAPM pain treatment guidelines. http://www.painmed.org/library/clinical-guidelines. Accessed May, 2020.

American Psychiatric Association. *Diagnostic and Statistical Manual of Mental Disorders*. 5th ed. Washington, DC: American Psychiatric Association, 2013.

American Society of Addiction Medicine. Definition of addiction. www.asam.org/resources/definition-of-addiction. Published 2019. Accessed January 4, 2019.

Azizi F, Vagenakis AG, Longcope C, Ingbar SH, Braverman LE. Decreased serum testosterone concentration in male heroin and methadone addicts. *Steroids*. 1973;22:467–472.

The ASAM Criteria. Treatment Criteria for Addictive, Substance-Related, and Co-Occurring Conditions. David Mee-Lee (ed.). American Society of Addiction Medicine. 3rd ed. Rockville, MD: 2013.

Barry DT, Irwin KS, Jones S, et al. Opioids, chronic pain, and addiction in primary care. *J Pain*. 2010;11(12):1442–1450.

Batki SL, Kauffman JF, Marion R, Parrino MW, Woody GE. *Medication-Assisted Treatment for Opioid Addiction in Opioid Treatment Programs*. Treatment Improvement Protocol (TIP) Series 43. DHHS Publication No. (SMA) 05-4048. Rockville, MD: Substance Abuse and Mental Health Services Administration; 2005

Beauchamp GA, Winstanley EL, Ryan SA, Lyons MS. Moving beyond misuse and diversion: the urgent need to consider the role of iatrogenic addiction in the current opioid epidemic. *Am J Public Health*. 2014;104(11):2023–2029.

Chang Y, Compton P. Management of chronic pain with chronic opioid therapy in patients with substance use disorders. *Addict Sci Clin Pract*. 2013;8(21):1–12.

Compton P, Charuvastra VC, Kintaudi K, Ling W. Pain responses in methadone-maintained opioid abusers. *J Pain Symptom Manage*. 2000;20(4):237–245.

Dunbar SA, Katz NP. Chronic opioid therapy for nonmalignant pain in patients with a history of substance abuse: report of 20 cases. *J Pain Symptom Manage*. 1996;11:163–171.

Eisenberg E, Suzan E, Pud D. Opioid-induced hyperalgesia (OIH): a real clinical problem or just an experimental phenomenon? *J Pain Symp Manag*. 2015;49(3):632–636.

Federation of State Medical Boards. Guidelines for the chronic use of opioid analgesics. https://www.fsmb.org/siteassets/advocacy/policies/opioid_guidelines_as_adopted_april-2017_final.pdf. Published April 2017. Accessed May, 2020.

Fraser LA, Morrison D, Morley-Forster P, et al. Oral opioids for chronic noncancer pain: higher prevalence of hypogonadism in men than in women. *Exp Clin Endocrinol Diabetes*. 2009;117:38–43.

Katz, NP, Adams, EH. Benneyan, JC. Foundations of opioid risk management. *Clin J Pain*. 2007;23(2):103–118.

Kumar P, Kumar N, Thakur DS, Patidar A. Male hypogonadism: symptoms and treatment. *J Adv Pharm Technol Res*. 2010;1(3):297–301.

Prater CD, Zylstra RG, Miller KE. Successful pain management for the recovering addicted patient. *Primary Car Companion J Clin Psychiatry*. 2002;4(4):124-131.

Suboxone. *Drugs.com*. www.drugs.com/pro/suboxone.html. Accessed January 4, 2019.

Substance Abuse and Mental Health Services Administration, US Department of Health and Human Services. *The facts about buprenorphine for treatment of opioid addiction*. Washington, DC: US Department of Health and Human Services; 2009.

Substance Abuse and Mental Health Services Administration, US Department of Health and Human Services. *Clinical guidelines for the use of buprenorphine in the treatment of opioid addiction*. Treatment Improvement Protocol (TIP) Series 40. DHHS Publication No. (SMA) 04–3939. Rockville, MD: US Department of Health and Human Services; 2004.

Volkow V, Friden TR, Hyde PS, Cha SS, Medication-assisted therapies: tackling the opioid-overdose epidemic. *N Engl J Med*. 2014;370:2063–2066.

Webster LR, Webster RM. Predicting aberrant behaviors in opioid-treated patients: preliminary validation of the Opioid Risk Tool. *Pain Med*. 2005;6(6):432–442.

8 Psychologically Immobilized and Functionally Paralyzed

Robert is a 55-year-old male presenting with a history of neck and low-back pain. He was initially injured on the job, recovered, and returned to work. Within a year he was re-injured, resulting in surgery to his low back. Recovery was protracted, and his surgeon cautioned Robert about any heavy lifting. As a consequence, he has developed a morbid fear of re-injury. He is hesitant to engage in almost any activity. According to his wife, he has become a "couch potato." He justifies his activity avoidance by noting that he was the one who suffered through surgery and has no intention of doing it again. The situation has begun to threaten the marriage. His adult kids fuss at, and resent, his lack of involvement with the grandchildren. He is more than willing to increase his activity, if he can get enough medicine to prevent the pain.

What do you do now?

BACKGROUND

Robert's case is probably more the norm then exception. He displays what pain clinicians refer to as *kinesiophobia* (KP). KP is defined as an irrational, weakening, and devastating fear of movement and activity stemming from the belief of fragility and susceptibility to injury (Kori et al, 1990). Following an injury, especially one that results in surgery, persistent pain, and apparent physical limitations, many patients develop a morbid fear of re-injury or increased pain. This fear can reach paralytic proportions, all but incapacitating, mentally and physically, the patient. KP has also been associated with the development of allodynia (pain sensitivity to previously nonpainful stimuli) in migraine sufferers (Benatto et al, 2019).

KP can have its origins in thoughts and experiences that predate actual injury. Two concepts are relevant: resilience and salience. In physics, *resilience* is the ability of an elastic material to absorb energy and release that energy as it springs back to its original shape. Psychologically, resilience is that quality that allows some people to be knocked down by life and rebound back. Resilient individuals (i) experience only transient and mild disruptions in functioning; (ii) dysregulation and variability in emotional/physical well-being is relatively brief and does not significantly impede their ability to function; and (iii) continue to fulfill personal/social responsibilities and maintain a capacity for generative experiences (Bonanno et al, 2005). *Salience* is the quality of being noticeable or standing out. Salient events attract attention and are meaningful or behaviorally relevant. Patients with histories of recovery from injury are likely to have developed coping skills, psychologically and physically, that keep pain in perspective, tend to minimize pain salience, and inoculate them against conditions like KP.

Figure 8.1 illustrates the process associated with KP. It is initiated by a pain-causing injury. The motivated, resilient patient responds to the pain of the injury or associated recovery (ie, physical rehabilitation) with an appropriate (adaptive) level of fear. They understand it to be part of the recovery process. They approach their rehabilitation with the expectation of improvement, utilize modalities (eg, heat, ice, etc.), and low-level analgesics to manage the pain. This is commonly observed in athletes.

Others respond to pain with catastrophic thoughts, imaging the worse. Pain represents injury/damage and is to be avoided. These thoughts persist,

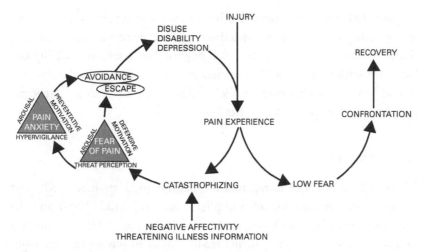

FIGURE 8.1 Fear-Avoidance Model.

Adopted from: Leeuw M, Goossens EJB, Linton S, Crombez G, Boersma K, Vlaeyen J, The fear-avoidance model of musculoskeletal pain: current state of scientific evidence, *J Behav Med.* 30(1):77–94.

despite reassurance that pain is part of the recovery process. The fear of pain becomes coupled with pain anxiety. This is not unlike the child who, after being scared by a dog, fears all dogs and sometimes all animals. The mere prospect of contact evokes fear and avoidance behavior. The patient with chronic pain finds that avoiding certain activities/movements protects them from the pain, albeit temporarily. They quickly learn to escape/terminate any such activities. However, by virtue of the associated inactivity, they become very physically deconditioned and weak with shortened muscles, such that almost any movement now evokes pain. This deconditioning is often associated with inflammation, which prompts greater pain intensity and sensitivity.

The persistent fear of pain, enhanced by exaggerated and maladaptive thoughts, provokes a high level of pain vigilance (salience). This process is perpetuated and reinforced by the predictable appearance of pain with minimal activity. KP becomes more intractable in the presence of a reinforcing consequences (eg, attentive spouse, financial incentive, etc.). Conditioning theory accurately predicts that the mere thought of doing an activity (eg, household chore, eating out, walking, exercise, etc.) can produce a sense of pain. This has been confirmed by functional magnetic resonance imaging studies showing increased activity in areas of the brain referred to as the pain matrix in response to such thoughts. The resultant disability can have devastating emotional consequences. Some seek out medication (ie, opioids) to cope. Other may use illicit drugs or alcohol. Reduced participation in the marriage and family has led to divorce.

ASSESSMENT

There are several questionnaire that can be used to detect KP. The Tampa Scale for Kinesiophobia (Miller, Kori, and Todd, 1991) and the Fear Avoidance Beliefs Questionnaire (Waddell et al, 1993) are but two examples. However, many patients readily admit to staying in their night clothes and not leaving the house for days on end secondary to their pain. They avoid household chores and only go places if escape is easy to arrange. They receive a good deal of assistance from others. Some express a sense of helplessness; others appear to have adapted and accepted. Some will protest their poor quality of life and profess a desire to be more active. However, they defer responsibility to the medical system, often saying to clinicians, "You have to do something."

The most extreme cases present to the office using assistive devices, which may not be necessary, and accompanied by a significant other. They have a very slow, gingerly gait and may have a back brace or cushion of some type. They are slow getting up and down from a sedated position and frequently adjust their position. Importantly, the neurological examination is generally unremarkable, as are radiological studies. There is hypersensitivity to palpation, even outside the areas of pain. Their facial expression may be inconsistent with their pain rating. At times, it can be difficult to differentiate KP form malingering or symptom exaggeration.

TREATMENT

No single type, combination, or amount of medication will resolve KP. Indeed, it may reinforce it. KP is a psychological problem. Although it manifests itself in the patient's numerical pain rating (NPR), most experienced clinicians recognize there is little correlation between NPR and function. However, because of the ease with which it can be obtained, a reduction is NPR is a metric for effective treatment. It is this unfounded emphasis on the NPR that has contributed to the opioid crisis: "The root problem may be neither the high risk or the low efficacy of long term opioid therapy but rather an improper focus on reducing pain intensity" (Sullivan and Ballantyne, 2016, p. 67). Indeed, a study by Backonja and Farrar (2015) reported that the most common reason to obtaining an NRP was to justify the prescribing of analgesics. In addition, there is no correlation between levels of pain and patient satisfaction with treatment (Comley and DeMeyer, 2001). Assuming pain is the reason for inactivity, one could identify three or so functional goals and use analgesics only to the extent that functioning improves.

Treatment of KP involves addressing the patient's feelings, thoughts, and behaviors. Box 8.1 summarizes therapeutics procedures for each. In general, motivation interviewing is designed to discover how prepared the patients is to accepting and implementing changes (Rollinick et al, 2008). The patient is encouraged to identify the pros and cons so as to better process and ultimately resolve the conflict between them. Although empathizing with the patient, the clinician encourages them to take steps toward making a change. This can involve differentiating (i) hurt (pain) and harm, (ii) the long-term negative consequences of inactivity, and (iii) the positive consequences of exercise and increased activity. The steps involved toward building motivation for change are list in Box 8.1.

This is not unlike helping someone to realize the benefits of not smoking or weight loss. Some simply will not get it. Stick with them; time may or

TABLE 8.1 **Therapeutic Targets and Intervention**

Therapeutic Target	Intervention
Activity avoidance; anticipatory pain	Operant conditioning (ie, graded exercise program, desensitization, education)
Cognitive distortions (eg, maladaptive cognitive-behavioral therapy (acceptance therapy, beliefs, expectations, and/or coping)	Cognitive restructuring, motivational interviewing, education
Anxiety, fear, somatic hypervigilance	Relaxation training; self-hypnosis; desensitization; education

Adapted from Gatchel RJ, Turk DC, eds. *Psychological Approaches to Pain Management: A Practitioner's Handbook*. New York, NY, Guilford Press, 1996. A description of each intervention can be found here as well.

may not help. Be careful not to perpetuate their sedentary style via drugs. Table 8.1 provides some suggestions for interventions.

A functionally oriented musculoskeletal therapist can assess the patient and design a graded exercise program. Ideally, this should be done under supervision in a clinic setting but can be the patient can be given a home-exercise-program. Most therapists can determine on follow-up if the patient is compliant. Many on Medicare may qualify for the Silver Sneakers program (www.sliversneakers.com) wherein their insurance plan will cover the fee to join a local exercise facility. This removes a major barrier. If available, patients should be encouraged to join a facility with a heated indoor pool. An aquatics program involving simply moving about in the water several times a week is a good starting place for almost anyone. The buoyancy of the water renders the patient 40% lighter while the warmth can relax the muscles.

Modalities, medication, interventional therapy, etc. can be made contingent upon compliance. Some clinicians work harder to get the patient better than the patient does. "Feel good" treatments should be a reward and not a replacement for patient involvement. However draconian this may sound, it works! This process of gradual desensitization may take time, perhaps a year or so, but it pays dividends.

There is always a plethora of maladaptive thoughts associated with KP: "There is no way I can tolerate this"; "If I try to do anything, I will be in bed for days"; "I cannot do this without more medication"; "I know my body, and what is best"; "I am not going to run the risk of injury and another surgery"; "If you had my pain, you would understand." Cognitive restructuring is a psychotherapeutic process of learning to identify and dispute irrational or maladaptive thoughts known as cognitive distortions, such as all-or-nothing thinking (splitting), magical thinking, overgeneralization, magnification, and emotional reasoning.

Cognitive-behavioral therapy combines cognitive therapy (ie, cognitive restructuring with behavior therapy) by identifying faulty or maladaptive patterns of thinking, emotional response, or behavior and substituting them with desirable patterns of thinking, emotional response, or behavior. Although formally done by pain psychologist, do not underestimate your ability to influence your patient's thoughts and perceptions. Clinicians, especially surgeons, are seen by patients as authoritative. Their comments can elicit fear or confidence. The catastrophizing and fearful patient will likely overgeneralize any cautionary statement. What is intended to minimize future injury can be incapacitating.

Pain associated with rehabilitation and life in general needs to put in context. The clinician can facilitate this by communicating with the surgeon and giving feedback to the patient and significant others. Introducing and reinforcing more adaptive pain coping skills such as positive self-statements, ignoring, goal-setting, diverting or redirecting attention, and reinterpreting. Oddly enough, grandchildren and pets tend to promote increased activity.

There is strong evidence that educating patients as to the neurophysiology and neurobiology of pain can positively impact pain, disability, catastrophizing, and physical performance (Lauw et al, 2011). Obtaining, reviewing, and interpreting radiology reports can be instructive. A patient may be told nothing is wrong—meaning there is no surgical lesion—or the damage is so extensive that surgery will not help. In both cases, clarification is needed to prevent an exaggerated interpretation of meaning of anatomical deformities.

- In general, chronic pain management should be rehabilitative versus palliative.
- Function trumps pain: improved quality of life/function produces greater satisfaction and long-term benefits than a simple reduction is pain rating score.
- Some patients are well-engrained in their sedentary life. They lack the necessity and motivation to change. Avoid the pit fall of "contributing by prescribing."
- Overcoming KP is a long-term process—in some cases, literally one step at a time.
- Addressing the patient's thoughts and motivation can be critical. Exercise can be good for what ails you.

Further Reading

Backonja M, Farrar JT. Are pain rating irrelevant? *Pain Med.* 2015;16:1247–1250.

Benatto MT, Bevilaqua-Grossi B, Carvalho GF, Bragatto MM, Pinheiro CF. Kinesiophobia is associated with migraine. *Pain Med.* 2019;20(4):846–851.

Bonanno GA, Rennicke C, Dekel S. Self-enhancement among high exposure survivors of the September 11th terrorist attack: resilience or social maladjustment? *J Person Soc Psychol.* 2005;88:984–998.

Comley AL, DeMeyer EJ. Assessing patient satisfaction with pain management through a continuous quality improvement effort. *Pain Symptom Manage.* 2001;21(1):27–40.

Kori SH, Miller RP, Todd DD. Kinesiophobia: a new view of chronic pain behavior. *Pain Manage.* 1990;3:35–43.

Louw A, Diener I, Butler DS, Puentedura MJ. The effect of neuroscience education on pain, disability, anxiety, and stress in chronic musculoskeletal pain. *Arch Phys Med Rehabil.* 2011;92:2041–2056.

Miller RP, Kori S, Todd D. The Tampa Scale: a measure of kinesiophobia. *Clin J Pain.* 1991;7(1):51–52.

Rollnick, S., Miller W., Butler, C. *Motivational Interviewing in Health Care: Helping Patients Change Behavior.* 2008. New York, NY: Guilford Press.

Sullivan M, Ballantyne J. Must we reduce pain intensity to treat chronic pain? *Pain.* 2016;157:65–69.

Waddell G, Newton M, Henderson I, Somerville D, Main CJ. A Fear-Avoidance Beliefs Questionnaire (FABQ) and the role of fear-avoidance beliefs in chronic low back pain and disability. *Pain.* 1993;52:157–168.

9 The "What If" and "Yes But" Syndrome

Sally is a 37-year-old female with a history of chronic widespread pain. She is relatively new to your practice. She does not make excessive demands for medication but always seems emotionally overwhelmed by her chronic pain. She finds it hard to discuss anything else. She worries about the significance of any change in her symptoms. She readily admits it is on her mind 24/7. She feels the situation is hopeless and that she is destiny to live in misery. Sally seems to shun any reinterpretation of her symptoms or encouragement. At time you wonder why she even returns to the clinic; but she does.

What would you do now?

BACKGROUND

The concept of catastrophizing emerged from the work of Albert Ellis in 1962 and Arron Beck in 1970s. Pain catastrophizing (PC) is conceptualized as a negative cognitive-affective response to anticipated or actual pain. PC involves magnification of negative consequences, persistent rumination, and feelings of hopelessness and helplessness regarding ones potential to effectively cope. The threat value of the painful event is magnified, and there is the perceived inability to inhibit pain-related thoughts in anticipation of, during, or following a painful encounter. Unfortunately, PC takes on the quality of a self-fulfilling prophecy. That is, the cognitive and emotional reaction does, indeed, enhance the effects of pain.

It is currently unclear if PC represents a trait (dispositional) or state (situational) characteristic. Regarding the former, initial conceptualizations of catastrophizing considered maladaptive thoughts to be latent and manifest following exposure to an appropriate cue. Some data suggest that state-related PC be may strongly correlated with pain related physiological and psychological/behavioral measures than trait-related PC. PC appears to intersect with pain anxiety, fear of pain, and pain helplessness, and to share some aspects of depression, anxiety, anxiety sensitivity, worry, and neuroticism.

Because patients that engage in PC tend to be overly dramatic and exaggerated, they can easily be confused with the patient with a hysterical personality style. However, the behavior of the patient with histrionic personality disorder (American Psychiatric Association, 2013) is more broad and all-encompassing (Box 9.1). It often involves dramatic behavior aimed at gaining the approval of others, flirtatious, emotional, seductive, or otherwise attention-seeking behavior. Indeed, they may engage in PC, but this is not the primary symptom.

Michael Sullivan and Robert R. Edwards have contributed heavily to contemporary studies on PC. PC appears to be a very robust concept and applicable to both acute and chronic pain. It has been found to correlate with pain outcome measures in the experimental and clinical settings involving various populations (eg, pain-free, normal, depressed, chronic pain, and arthritic patients). PC levels have been associated with postsurgical pain ratings and narcotic usage. One study found that preoperative PC levels predicted chronic postoperative (keen arthroplasty) pain at 24 months (Forsythe et al, 2008). In addition, PC has correlated with increased levels of interleukin-6, a pro-inflammatory substance associated with the onset and persistence of chronic pain (Edwards et al, 2008). PC has been shown to impact pain severity, pain-related activity interference, disability, depression, social support networks, and suicidal ideation. High PC levels tend to be found in patients with low self-efficacy regarding their ability to cope with pain, and high levels of dependency. Importantly, PC has been associated with reduced effectiveness of analgesics, especially opioids (for details, see Quartana et al, 2009; Edwards et al, 2008).

ASSESSMENT

The most common questionnaire used in the assessment of PC is the Pain Catastrophizing Scale (Sullivan et al, 1995; Box 9.2). It provides three subscales: helplessness, rumination, and magnification. Each of 13 items is scored on a 4-point scale (0 = not at all, 4 = all the time) for a total of 52 points. A score of 30 or more indicates clinical relevant PC. In recognition of the fact that PC usually occurs in a social context, Cano et al (2005) developed the Spouse/Significant Other Version of the PCS. This instrument assesses the impact on, and response tendencies of, significant others.

It is not difficult to recognize high PC in the clinic. They appear worried, anxious, emotional, and demanding. They express a sense of futility and, although not suicidal, bemoan their situation and are unsure how they can possibly live this way. They see their reaction as perfectly normal. It is important two distinguish PC from drug-seekers, whose sole purpose is to obtain more medication by convincing the clinician that the current dose is too low to manage their "horribly severe, debilitating, and all-consuming pain." Drug-seekers are likely to focus on the medication while the high PC patients focus on the pain, its effect, and their feelings of helplessness. Most certainly, PC can overlap with, and be a component of, depression. One should look for the typical signs of depression including anhedonia, changes in appetite/weight, insomnia, loss of energy, irritability, problems concentrating, and suicidal thoughts (see Box 1.2 in Chapter 1 of this volume).

TREATMENT

Treatment studies in the area of PC involving chronic noncancer pain populations have focused largely on musculoskeletal low back pain, neck pain, osteoarthritis, fibromyalgia, neuropathic pain, and perioperative pain for keen surgery (for details, see Schutze et al, 2018). The treatments of choice have been cognitive-behavioral therapy (CBT), acceptance and commitment therapy (ACT), and multimodal treatment combining CBT and physical therapy (PT). (These therapies are reviewed in detail in the Chapter 21 of this volume.) In general, CBT focuses on helping the patient to recognize, evaluate, and modify maladaptive pain-related thoughts, emotions, and behaviors. ACT, however, is based on the assumption that although pain hurts, it is the struggle with pain that causes suffering and intensifies the negative consequences of painful events. ACT encourages the development of awareness and a nonjudgmental acceptance of chronic pain while emphasizing the identification and commitment to valued goals and activities.

Multimodal therapy incorporates CBT/ACT with PT. Adding PT, especially in the form of functional restoration and/or graded in vivo exercise (ie, exercise that demands gradually increased) can be particularly helpful and has been shown to be superior to CBT or ACT alone. Although exercise does not directly target negative thinking associated with PC, including a well-designed exercise routine may (i) help to shift attention away from ruminating about pain, (ii) provide a demonstration that activity need not produce catastrophic outcomes, (iii) facilitates cognitive restructuring by providing disconfirmatory evidence, (iv) increase the use of exercise as a self-management tool, and (v) increase self-efficacy and reduces the sense of helplessness. A recent review involving 79 studies (9,914 total participants) found that the magnitude of the effects of treatment was "medium" in general and of questionable clinical significance. However, when applied to those with high levels of PC, the effects were larger and more consistent. Multimodal treatment yielded the strongest effects overall.

Research efforts are underway by the team at Sanford University to explore the effects of a single session of therapy for PC. It may be that simply having the patient complete the PCS, followed by a brief discussion of how the use of such exaggerated terms can intensify pain and suggesting more appropriate ones would suffice. One could use the example of the effect of how an overreactive versus calm parental response can influence a child's reactions.

Caution should be exercised regarding the use of medication. Although these patients can seem very anxious and distraught, the use of psychotropic and benzodiazepines may be counterproductive. Likewise, the use of analgesics in the presence of increased complaints of pain will only serve to exacerbate the problem. The fundamental antagonist are (i) cognitive processes, (ii) low self-efficacy, and (iii) limited coping skills. Whenever possible, involving a pain-oriented psychologist, if only for a few sessions, can be very beneficial.

Be careful not to marginalize or dismiss the patient's concerns. Rather, help to clarify the potentially negative impact of their PC. Introducing more realistic and productive self-statements, especially support by objective testing can be useful. For example, helping the patient understand that the presence of arthritic changes does not mean they have to abandon valued activities but may require some adaptation, which is ultimately needed as a result of the aging process anyway.

KEY POINTS TO REMEMBER

- The mechanisms by which PC exerts its effects appear to include cognitive-attentional processes, social interactions, and neural pain-modulatory systems.
- PC may be causally related to the onset and maintenance of persistent pain syndromes including postsurgical neuropathic pain, low back pain, and neck/shoulder pain.
- PC reduces the analgesic effect of pain medicine, especially opioids.
- PC has been associated with a number of pain-related outcomes, including acute and chronic pain severity, altered central nervous system pain processing (eg, diminished endogenous pain inhibition), exaggerated healthcare utilization, postsurgical pain outcomes and disability, and pain-related activity interference.
- Patient with high scores of PC attend most readily to pain-related stimuli and have a particularly pronounced inability to disengage cognitive resources from such stimuli.

- PC can exert significant, and potentially deleterious, effects on a patient's support network. It has been associated with punishing responses from the spouse/significant other.
- PC is associated with altered hypothalamic pituitary responses to pain and amplified activation in neural regions implicated in processing and regulation of affective components of pain (eg, anterior cingulate cortex).
- Assess and address early on in treatment.

Further Reading

Beck AT. *Cognitive Therapy of Depression*. New York: Guilford Press; 1979.

Cano A, Leonard MT, Franz A. The Significant Other Version of the Pain Catastrophizing Scale (PCS-S): preliminary validation. *Pain*. 2005;119(1–3):26–37.

Edwards RR, Kronfli T, Haythornthwaite JA, Smith MT, McGuire L, Page GG. Association of catastrophizing with interleukin-6 responses to acute pain. *Pain*. 2008;140(1):135–144.

Ellis A. *Reason and Emotion in Psychotherapy*. New York, NY: L. Stuart; 1962.

Forsythe ME, Dunbar MJ, Hennigar AW, Sullivan MJ, Gross M. Prospective relation between catastrophizing and residual pain following knee arthroplasty: two-year follow-up. *Pain Res Manag*. 2008;13(4):335–341.

Quartana PJ, Campbell CM, Edwards RR. Pain catastrophizing: a critical review. *Expert Rev Neurother*. 2009;9(5):745–758.

Rosentiel AK, Keefe FJ. The use of coping strategies in chronic low back pain patients: relationship to patient characteristics and current adjustment. *Pain*. 1983;17:33–44.

Schütze R, Rees C, Smith A, Slater H, Campbell JM, O'Sullivan P. How can we best reduce pain catastrophizing in adults with chronic non-cancer pain? A systematic review and meta-analysis. *J Pain*. 2018;19(3):233–256.

Sullivan MJL, Bishop SR, Pivik J. The pain catastrophizing scale: development and validation. *Psychol Assess*. 1995;7(4):524–532.

10 The Patient Who Remembers Tomorrow

Helen is a 72-year-old female seen along with her sister. When asked, Helen was unsure who referred her or why she was referred. Brief screening showed that she could recall six digits forward. She thought she had been married twice and was still married but, in fact, had been married four times and was divorced. She reported pain in her left thigh but was very vague regarding its qualitative and quantitative characteristics. When her sister stated her pain was detected because she would complain, the patient seemed surprised and resentful. She continues to be fairly functional and independent in personal care. Helen has been through medication management, interventional therapy, and physical therapy, some of which she could not recall, without any apparent benefit. Spinal cord stimulation was being considered. The family seems more concerned than patient about her pain.

What do you do now?

BACKGROUND

This section will focus on cognitive dysfunction as a result of neurological conditions such as dementia and Alzheimer's disease (AD). We will not be considering cognitive dysfunction, which is transient (eg, related to insomnia, intoxication, etc.). We will address the ambulatory patient the clinician is likely to see in the office setting rather than those in a facility and/ or requiring full-time care.

Dementia is defined as a *"clinical syndrome* due to disease of the brain, usually of a progressive nature, which leads to disturbances of multiple higher cortical functions, including memory, thinking, orientation, comprehension, calculation, learning capacity, language, and judgment" (World Health Organization, 2010, Emphasis added, p. 8). Its symptoms are common to several brain diseases including AD, vascular dementia, Parkinson's disease, dementia, Huntington's disease dementia, frontotemporal dementia, and Wernicke-Korsakoff syndrome. These neurodegenerative disorders can result in a progressive and irreversible loss of neurons and brain functioning. It is fairly common to witness a combination of gray matter atrophy and white matter lesions. These changes are associated with a variety of functional, emotional, and behavioral consequences (see Table 10.1).

Approximately 50% of patients with dementia experiences pain (Corbett et al, 2012); 32% home-dwelling patients, and 60% of those in a nursing home. The prevalence of pain is age-related involving 72% above the age of 85 years. Nearly 40% of patients with PD have pain secondary to their underlying movement disorder. Those with dementia and pain had a 9.2%

TABLE 10.1 **Levels of Dementia**

Mild	Moderate	Severe	Terminal
Impaired memory	Confused	Resistiveness	Bedfast
Personality changes	Agitation	Incontinence	Mute
Spatial disorientation	Insomnia	Eating difficulties	Frequent infections
Social withdrawal	Aphasia	Motor impairment	Dysphasia
Decreased insight	Apraxia	Inability to smile	

more rapid decline in memory compared to those without pain. In addition, the probability of dementia increased 7.7% and occurred at an earlier age in people who had persistent pain compared with those that had none (Whitlock et al, 2017). Rates were comparable among those treated with opioids versus nonsteroidal anti-inflammatory drugs (NSAIDs; Dublin et al, 2015).

The medial pain system appears to be more compromised then the lateral system. Therefore, the cognitive-evaluative and motivational-affective aspects of pain are more affected than the sensory-discriminative aspects. Karp et al (2008) hypothesized the existence of a diminished response to the stress associated with aging and cognitive dysfunction, which suppresses the otherwise strong homeostatic drive associated with pain. This results in a state of *homeostenosis* (constriction of an aging individual's ability to effectively respond to stress because of diminished biological, psychological, and social reserves).

However, some studies suggest that pain processing, pain reflexes, and facial responses to noxious stimuli are not only maintained but, indeed, may be enhanced in patients with AD. There appears to be greater activation of the striatum in response to painful stimuli in those with mild to moderate AD (Acterberg et al, 2013). Functional connectivity between the cortical and subcortical brain regions also appeared enhanced in patients with AD.

ASSESSMENT

Assessment of pain in people with dementia is particularly challenging due to the loss of communication ability limiting the subjective reporting of pain normally anticipated in cognitively healthy adults. Interestingly, sensory and affective components of pain can be differentially expressed in the face, with sensory aspects shown by movements around the eyes, and affective aspects depicted by movements of the eyebrows and the upper lip. Symptoms can very day to day and, at times, within the day (eg, sundowners syndrome), further complicating assessment. Some of the more common and revealing behaviors associated with pain are shown in Box 10.1. Observations by caregivers or persons having regular contact with the patient are often necessary.

> **BOX 10.1 Common Pain Behaviors in Cognitively Impaired Elderly Persons**
>
> *Facial expressions*: Slight frown, sad, frightened face, grimacing, wrinkled forehead, closed or tightened eyes, distorted expression, rapid blinking, inexpressive
>
> *Verbalizations/vocalizations*: Sighing, moaning, groaning, grunting, chanting, calling out, noisy breathing, asking for help, verbally abusive
>
> *Body movements*: Rigid, tense body posture, guarding, fidgeting, increased pacing, rocking, restricted movement, gait or mobility changes
>
> *Changes in interpersonal interactions*: Aggressive, combative, resisting care, decreased social interactions, socially inappropriate, disruptive, withdrawn
>
> *Changes in activity patterns or routines*: Refusing food, appetite change, increase in rest periods, sleep, rest pattern changes, increased wandering
>
> *Mental status changes*: Crying or tears, increased confusion, irritability or distress
>
> Free evidence-based tools and best practices for nurses, who work in nursing homes, are available through www.geriatricpain.org.
> From AGS Panel on Persistent Pain in Older Persons, The management of persistent pain in older persons. *J Am Geriatr Soc.* 2002;50(Suppl 6):S205–S224.

TREATMENT

Significant treatment disparities exist. One studied showed patients with dementia were prescribed one third the amount of morphine compared to those without dementia, and 76% had no standing order for postoperative analgesia (Morrison and Siu, 2000). Only 33% of patients with AD got appropriate analgesia versus 64% patients without AD, regardless of the medication (opioid, automatic positive airway pressure, or NSAID), despite the treating clinicians judging the two groups as equivalent in their pain (Scherder and Bouma, 1997). The discussion of treatment will be divided to several sections: recognition, management, and pharmacology.

Recognition. Some patients are unaware, or in denial, of their cognitive deficits. They interpret their ability to function day-to-day as evidence of intact mental functioning and decision-making capability. Some level of neurocognitive testing and a family involvement may be necessary to convince the patient of their status. Patients loathe the idea of giving up any degree of independence. Highlighting the risk to themselves and others may help.

Management. Using family members to monitor medication-taking can elicit a variety of responses depending upon the nature of the patient–family relationship. Reaction can range for acceptance and appreciation to anger, belligerence, rebellion, and defiance. In the end, the clinician must do what must be done to protect the patient. Automated dispensers (see www.MedReady-Medication-Dispenser-Flashing), which can be loaded, secured, and programmed by the clinician (or designated staff), can be useful. These dispensers emit an audible cue signaling the availability of medication and limiting access until the appropriate time. The use of teletherapy or phone apps can facilitate oversight while minimizing cumbersome visits to the office, especially for those with mobility issues. Changes can occur rapidly and unpredictably. Therefore, frequent contact, at least monthly, is suggested. Symptoms, and thus the effects of medications, can vary day to day and within the day, and one should be careful about making knee-jerk treatment modifications. It is important to obtain an update medication list to review for drug–drug interactions. Be especially aware of herbal and dietary supplements.

Pharmacological. The effectiveness of opioid therapy can be influenced by the patient's neurocognitive status. Patients with AD have a fairly normal response to sensory stimuli (Benedetti et al, 2004, 2006) but lower pain intensity and pain-related affect compared to controls. Also, the placebo-related and expectation-related mechanisms appear to be compromised. Box 10.2 lists pain-related characteristics/behaviors often seen in patient with cognitive impairment.

By virtue of the diminished placebo response, the use of drugs with more salient drug onset cues (ie, short-acting) may be advisable. It is interesting that there is some evidence that low-dose opioids may help to control dementia-related agitation and impulsiveness (Brown, 2010, Love et al, 2009). Over-the-counter medications, NSAIDs, antidepressants, muscle relaxers, and anti-epileptic drugs may have a role. At times, it is the simple act of taking something (self-administration cues) that produces relief. The pharmacokinetics and pharmacodynamics establish via short-term Phase III trials may not be applicable.

Other medical conditions (eg, gastrointestinal, cardiac, hepatic, and/or renal dysfunction) may contraindicate the use of long-activating or sustained-release preparations. Topical preparations can be useful for localized pain such as arthritic joints. Use of interventional and neuromodulation therapy should be approached with caution. Despite a successful pre-implant trial, the benefits can dissipate quickly. Some patients eventually find implanted devices very unsettling.

One of the most comprehensive guidelines on the medication management of pain in the elderly was authored by a panel from the American Geriatrics Society (American Geriatrics Society Panel on Pharmacological Management of Persistent Pain in Older Persons, 2009). Following is a summary of recommendations (please review these guidelines for details).

Dosing: Start at 30% to 50% of the recommended starting dose and titrated upward in 25% increments for comfort and side effect tolerance.

Acetaminophen: Initiate treatment with acetaminophen for chronic musculoskeletal pain because of its relatively benign side effect profile as long as the recommended daily dose is not exceeded 2000 mg/day.

NSAIDs: Can follow acetaminophen in the treatment of chronic musculoskeletal pain. NSAIDs often provide more analgesia for bone pain than other analgesics.

Opioids: Opioid analgesics can play a major role in the treatment of moderate to severe acute and cancer-related pain. Their use in patients of any age with chronic noncancer pain still remains controversial because of their side effects. Special caution needs to be taken when using methadone. It can be an excellent analgesic, but because its analgesic effect lasts only 6 to 8 hours, which is much shorter than its half-life of 16 to 30 hours, metabolites can accumulate and cause significant side effects. Opioids with no active metabolites are a better choice in older adults.

Anticonvulsants: Many anticonvulsants appear to provide analgesia; most commonly used are pregabalin and gabapentin.

Antidepressants: Tricyclic antidepressants and serotonin-norepinephrine reuptake inhibitors (eg, duloxetine and venlafaxine) have been shown to have analgesic properties. However, TCAs have not been approved as analgesics by the US Food and Drug Administration.

Topical: Lidocaine 5% patch and capsaicin and two topical analgesics, in addition to the topical NSAIDS, are worth considering:

Adjunctive/nonpharmacological therapies: Physical therapy can be very useful, especially for patients who have a pain-causing disease or injury that resulted in reduced activity levels leading to decreased activity tolerance. A home-based exercise program can maintain muscle strength and provide as element of distraction. Many community facility have suitable exercise programs, including aquatics therapy, and add an element of socialization. Modality therapies, transcutaneous electrical nerve stimulation (TENS), and massage can be considered. TENS can be used at home. It can provide relief but can also be prophylactic prior to patients engaging in activities, which they find difficult to avoid, such as sitting in a car for an extended period. For patients with a pacemakers, the use of TENS should cleared by their cardiologist. Occupational therapy can assist patients in performing activities of daily living and aid them in finding alternative, less painful ways to do these activities. Assessing the risk of falling and use of mobility aids can prevent further injury and pain. Psychotherapeutic techniques can help patients cope with chronic pain and potentially reduce the level of pain. These techniques are also beneficial when comorbid depression and pain are present. They can help to modulate agitated and impulsive behavior. Acupuncture can provide analgesia for a variety of chronic pain but the effect is likely to be short-lived.

KEY POINTS TO REMEMBER

- Assessment of pain in patients with dementia requires observational data.
- Older adults with dementia and chronic pain are not the same as younger patients with pain.
- Pain homeostenosis (less ability to respond effectively to the stress of chronic pain) can compromise assessment and effective treatment.
- Older adults with dementia and pain are more likely to lose function if there is a lack of timely intervention.
- Dementia-related cognitive dysfunction is associated with neurological changes at the cortical level. Aspects of pain processing and awareness involve subcortical structures.
- Treatment of depression in patients with dementia can have a significant impact on the pain.
- Be sure to differentiate behavioral disturbances as a sign of a pain requiring pain management versus psychiatric disorder requiring sedation. The sedated patient may still be in pain.
- Minimize polypharmacology.

Further Reading

Achterberg WP, Pieper MJC, van Dalen-Kok AH, et al. Pain management in patients with dementia. *Clin Interv Aging.* 2013;8:1471–1482.

American Geriatrics Society Panel on Pharmacological Management of Persistent Pain in Older Persons. Pharmacological management of persistent pain in older persons. *J Am Geriatr Soc.* 2009;57(8):1331–1346.

AGS Panel on Persistent Pain in Older Persons. The management of persistent pain in older persons. *J Am Geriatr Soc.* 2002;50(Suppl 6):S205–S224.

Benedetti F, Arduino C, Vighetti S. Pain reactivity in Alzheimer patients with different degrees of cognitive impairment and brain electrical activity deterioration. *Pain.* 2004;111:22–29.

Benedetti F, Arduino C, Costa S, et al. Loss of expectation-related mechanisms
in Alzheimer's disease makes analgesic therapies less effective. *Pain.*
2006;121:133–144.

Brown R. Broadening the search for safe treatments in dementia agitation a possible
role for low-dose opioids? *Int J Geriatr Psychiatry.* 2010;25:1085–1086.

Corbett A, Husebo B, Malcangio M, et al. Assessment and treatment of pain in people
with dementia. *Nat Rev Neurol.* 2012;8(5):264–274.

Dublin S, Walker RL, Gray SL, et al. Prescription opioids and risk of dementia
or cognitive decline: a prospective cohort study. *J Am Geriatr Soc.*
2015;63(8):1519–1526.

Karp JF, Shega JW, Morone NE, Weiner DK. Advances in understanding the
mechanisms and management of persistent pain in older adults. *Br J Anaesth.*
2008;101:111–120.

Love TM, Stohler CS, Zubieta JK. Positron emission tomography measures of
endogenous opioid neurotransmission and impulsiveness traits in humans.
Arch Gen Psychiatry. 2009;66:1124–1134.

Morrison RS, Siu AL. A comparison of pain and its treatment in advanced dementia
and cognitively intact patients with hip fracture. *J Pain Symptom Manage.*
2000;19(2):40–48.

Scherder EJ, Bouma A. Is decreased use of analgesics in Alzheimer disease due
to a change in the affective component of pain? *Alzheimer Dis Assoc Disord.*
1997;11:171–174.

Whitlock EL, Diaz-Ramirez LG, Glymour AM, Boscardin WJ, Covinsky KE, Smith AK.
Persistent pain was associated with accelerated memory decline and increased
probability of dementia: association between persistent pain and memory
decline and dementia in a longitudinal cohort of elders. *JAMA Intern Med.*
2017;177(8):1146–1153. doi:10.1001/jamainternmed.2017.1622

World Health Organization. *International Statistical Classification of Diseases
and Related Health Problems.* 10th rev. Geneva, Switzerland: World Health
Organization; 2010.

11 Please, Find It and Fix It

Mark is a 42-year-old male with a history of an on-the-job injury resulting in surgery to his to low back. He feels the outcome was not what he expected. He continues to have pain in a similar area. The numbness in his leg is better but not totally gone. He does not feel he can return to work or have a normal life in this condition. His surgeon has released him and reassured him that his symptoms are not unusual, and there is no indication of a further problem. He presents insisting that "something is wrong; the cause needs to be found; and its needs to be fixed. That is all I need!"

What do you do now?

BACKGROUND

The term "somatization disorder" (aka Briquet's syndrome) was used to refer to a mental disorder characterized by recurring, multiple, and current clinically significant complaints about somatic symptoms. A physical source or cause for the complaints could not be found resulting in the phrase "medically unexplained symptom(s)." Thus, the patient was thought to have a mental disorder and/or symptoms caused by some psychological problem. This engendered, and was an outgrowth of, a long-standing debate relating to the term "psychogenic pain," which was contrasted with "real" or physically based pain. Advancements in diagnostic technology and our understanding of chronic pain (neurophysiological, genetic, psychological factors) has been accompanied by some much-needed updating of these concepts (see Chapter 20 of this volume).

Somatization disorder, hypochondriasis, pain disorder, undifferentiated somatoform disorder and the phrase "medically unexplained symptom," previously appearing in the fourth edition of the *Diagnostic and Statistical Manual of Mental Disorders* (American Psychiatric Association, 1995) have been eliminated in the fifth edition (American Psychiatric Association, 2013) and replaced by somatic symptom disorder (SSD; Box 11.1). SSD is characterized by multiple, recurring physical complaints (eg, headaches, dizziness, chest pain, abdominal pain, limb pain, etc.), which may be difficult

---

BOX 11.1 **Criteria for Somatic Symptom Disorder**

A. One or more somatic symptoms that are distressing or result in significant disruption of daily life
B. Excessive thoughts, feelings, or behaviors related to the somatic symptoms or associated health concerns as manifested by at least one of the following
   1. Disproportionate and persistent thoughts about the seriousness of one's symptoms
   2. Persistently high level of anxiety about health or symptoms
   3. Excessive time & energy devoted to these symptoms or health concerns

Source: American Psychiatric Association. *Diagnostic and Statistical Manual of Mental Disorders*. 5th ed. Washington, DC: American Psychiatric Association; 2013.

to link to an identifiable medical condition. The SSD category include illness anxiety disorder (hypochondriasis), conversion disorder, psychological factors affecting other medical conditions, and factitious disorder. The latter refers to a situation wherein the symptoms are intentionally produced on one self or another.

SSD is based on the degree to which a person's thoughts, feelings, and behavior about their somatic symptoms are considered excessive and disruptive. Usually, the problem has existed for six months or more and is associated with disproportionate and persistent thoughts, feelings, and behaviors that border on an obsessive preoccupation with physical symptoms which interferes with normal life activities. However, the symptoms are not delusional, in the sense that they contradict or have no basis in reality. SSD is estimated to occur in 5% to 7% of the population with more in females than males. Those with SSD in childhood tend to continue to develop similar somatic symptoms in adulthood.

In Mark's case, he is convinced, based upon some persistent physical symptoms, that some serious physical abnormality has been overlooked. This is linked to an irrational fear of the potentially consequences and thus intensifies the salience of any physical symptoms. Simple reassurance is not likely to be sufficient to abate his concern.

Patients may become preoccupied with symptoms that can be attributed to normal bodily sensations. They engage in excessive worry and fear about the consequence of physical activity (see Chapter 8 of this volume). They often insist on repeated testing and examinations. Although they seek medical help and reassurance, the effects are short-lived. In the more severe cases, SSD may be accompanied by a severe depressive disorder and an increase risk for suicide Over 50% of depressed patients report somatic symptoms; many deny depression when questioned. Any suggestion of mental health services is rejected.

ASSESSMENT

It is important to distinguish SSD from a factitious disorder, wherein the patient causes physical damage to themselves or a proxy, and malingering wherein the complaints are designed to produce some desired external outcome such as disability, attention, avoidance of undesirable activity.

Parents with mood disorders and somatic symptoms tend to consult their primary care clinician on behalf of their children. The children may have more school absences for unexplained illnesses. Parental stress and mood disorders can manifest themselves in symptoms such as abdominal pain in children (Weisblatt et al, 2011). Social modeling, learned behavior, and beliefs can be key aspects of the environment created by the SSD patient and, in a sense, contaminate others in the family.

The current diagnostic criteria for SSD requires the presence of somatic symptoms (Criterion A) combined with a substantial impact of these symptoms on thoughts, emotions, and behaviors (Criterion B). Box 11.2 gives some suggestion for how to approach the assessment of someone suspected of SSD.

The Patient Health Questionnaire Somatic Symptom Severity Scale (PHQ-15) and the Somatic Symptom Scale (SSS-8) are commonly used assessment questionnaires. The PHQ-15 is a brief, self-administered questionnaire which can be used to assess somatic symptom severity (Kroenke et al, 2002). The PHQ-15 contains 15 items, which probe for somatic symptoms (eg, stomach pain, dizziness, etc.) present during the recent four-week period. The severity of the symptoms ("not bothered at all," "bothered a little," and "bothered a lot") is also assessed. The PHQ-15 scores of 5, 10, and 15 represent cut-off points for low, medium, and high somatic symptom severity, respectively (Kroenke et al, 2002). The SSS-8 is an 8-item

---

BOX 11.2 **Approach to the Patient with Multiple Somatic Symptoms**

Do a thorough history and detailed physical assessment
Rule out medical illness
Consider medication side effects
Identify ability to meet basic needs
Identify secondary gains
Identify ability to communicate emotional needs
Determine substance use
Build therapeutic alliance with the patient
Use screening tools appropriate for somatic symptom disorder

From Croicu C, Chwastiak L, Katon W. Approach to the patient with multiple somatic symptoms. *Med Clin N Am.* 2014;98(5):1070–1095.

patient-reported outcome measure of somatic symptom burden. It is the shortened version of the PHQ-15. The SSS-8 was developed with fifth edition of the *Diagnostic and Statistical Manual of Mental Disorders* (American Psychiatric Association, 2013) criteria in mind. The SSS-8 has a 5-point response option compared to three in the PHQ-15 and askes the patient to consider the previous seven versus 14-day period (Gierk et al, 2015).

Although the PHQ-15 and SSS-8 would be useful, the patient's presentation is often unmistakable and very revealing. What one is most likely to encounter is described in Table 11.1.

Asking the patient the reason(s) they doubt what they have been told, what tests they think would be conclusive, and what their approach would be if further treatment with potentially irreversible side effects were undertaken can provide some insight. Seeking input as to the difference between the patient's presurgical (treatment) expectations and the outcome could also provide a partial basis for their SSD. The impact of expectation

TABLE 11.1 **Clinical presentation of SSD**

Disproportionate and symptom-related thoughts	"This will never end." "How can I continue living with this." "I know my doctor says that everything is alright, but what if he has overlooked something." "There has got to be a reason I feel this way. I have to find a doctor who will help me." "This is ruining my life."
Persistent high level of health/symptom-related anxiety	Patient presents with anxiety, hopelessness, and despair. Patient is convicted something has been overlooked. Concerns may extend to symptoms beyond those related to the chronic pain (eg, cardiac).
Excessive time/energy spent on symptoms	Whenever the pain increase the patient seeks out a calm place, rests, and focuses his attention on his body—may take his own vital signs. Patient likely to engage in several consultations a month. The patient will ruminate about his symptoms, become easily distracted by them.

Adopted from Kleinstauber M, Rief W. Somatoform and related disorders: an update. *Psychiatric Times.* 2015;32(9).

management and a clearly articulate informed consent is often overlooked. The SSD patient may defer, claiming you are the doctor and should know the appropriate tests or may plead to have a previous test repeated at a different location or for some unique approach such as genetic testing. Their stated reassurance that they will be satisfied with the outcome should be taken lightly.

TREATMENT

SSD patients often seek help from a family physician believing they have a real, physical problem. Their care can be time-consuming and complicated. They may not trust the outcome of testing, no matter how sophisticated. Their response to treatment can be inconsistent and fraught with minor adverse reactions. Kleinstauber and Rief (2015) listed a number of strategies that should be avoided (Box 11.3).

Box 11.4 provides the recommended treatment strategies adopted from Croicu et al (2014) for the primary care setting.

In general, it is important to help the patient to understand that not every symptom can be explained. However, serious disease processes have been ruled out and you will monitor the situation. Emphasize the need to focus on improving function so as to decrease the burden on oneself and

---

BOX 11.3   Strategies to Be Avoided When Treating Patients With SSD

- Focus exclusively on a diagnosis.
- Always make a diagnosis.
- Dismiss the symptom as normal without addressing the patients concerns.
- Undertake excessive test without explaining the likelihood of a false-positive.
- Rely on drugs to treat the symptoms.
- Assume you know what the patients wants.
- Be judgmental and critical: attribute the patient's behavior to a single life event.
- Ignore or miss psychological cues.
- Assert psychosocial explanations which lead to defensiveness.
- Let your anxiety and uncertainty take over.

BOX 11.4 **Essential Treatment Approaches for Patients With Somatic Symptom Disorder**

- Schedule time-limited, regular appointments to address complaints.
- Educate patients how psychosocial stressors and symptoms interact.
- Educate the patient as to coping versus curing.
- Evaluate somatic symptom burden.
- Collaborate with the patient in setting treatment goals.
- Assess for comorbid psychiatric conditions (eg, depression, anxiety).
- If possible, treat comorbid psychiatric disorders (eg, tricyclic antidepressants, serotonin and noradrenalin reuptake inhibitor, serotonin reuptake inhibitors etc.; see Bleakley, 2013).
- When possible, consult with significant others.

Adapted from Croicu C, Chwastiak L, Katon W. Approach to the patient with multiple somatic symptoms. *Med Clin N Am*. 2014;98(5):1070–1095.

family. One should avoid comments such as "Your symptoms are all psychological" or "There is nothing wrong with you medically." Above all, avoid the merry-go-round of ordering unnecessary, repetitive, or invasive procedures/tests. The patient may reject the simplicity of your approach and choose to go elsewhere; so be it. In severe cases you may be threatened with medical/legal action if the problem worsens because you choose not to pursue it further. If the patient requests a referral to a specialist, have a release signed allowing communication with the specialist and requesting the results. Such a referral should not be initiated unless there is a valid medical reason.

Two forms of pharmacotherapy have been used with SSD: (i) somatic medication targeting the symptoms and (ii) the use of psychotropic medication (Mundt, 2013). Tricyclic antidepressants, serotonin reuptake inhibitors, serotonin and noradrenalin reuptake inhibitors, and atypical antipsychotics have been sued to target the symptoms of SSD. (Somashekar et al, 2013). The antidepressants may also help to reduce the depressive symptoms and hence somatic responses. Mood, fatigue, sleep, pain perception, gastrointestinal distress, and other somatic symptoms have been known to improve. The use of anti-anxiety medication (benzodiazepines) and opioids have a relative contraindication and should be considered for short-term use only. Agents such as Paxil® and BuSpar® can be used in place of benzodiazepines to treat anxiety.

When available mild to severe somatic complaints have responded to cognitive-behavioral therapy (CBT). CBT can influence the thought and behavior patterns, which, consciously or not, have triggered the physical symptom or the preoccupation with the symptom. The somatic complaints may been learned through a system of reinforcements and/or modeling (Shaw et al, 2011). Psychotherapy to deal with related family and social issues, and hypnosis for the development of coping skills. Family therapy may be necessary to (i) address the diverse possible causes of SSD, (ii) examine family relationships, and (iii) improve family support and functioning.

KEY POINTS TO REMEMBER

- Scheduling a regular visit with the patient reduces or eliminates unnecessary emergency department visits.
- Identifying risks such as childhood trauma can suggest screening for SSDs using appropriate assessment tools (PHQ-15 and SSS-8).
- Identifying, screening for, and treating common psychiatric comorbidities such as depression (PHQ-9) and anxiety (Generalized Anxiety Disorder-7) can decrease somatic symptom burden.
- Nonpharmacological interventions such as CBT has shown evidence in decreasing SSD.
- Therapeutic alliance with the patient with somatic complaints improves outcomes.
- Avoid the test–retest merry-go-round. Patience can be your ally.

Further Reading

American Psychiatric Association. *Diagnostic and Statistical Manual of Mental Disorders*. 4th ed. Washington, DC: American Psychiatric Association; 1995.

American Psychiatric Association. *Diagnostic and Statistical Manual of Mental Disorders*. 5th ed. Washington, DC: American Psychiatric Association; 2013.

Bleakley S. Review of the choice and use of antidepressant drugs. *Progress in Neurology and Psychiatry*. 2013;17:18–26.

Bøen H, Dalgard OS, Bjertness E. The importance of social support in the associations between psychological distress and somatic health problems and socio-economic factors among older adults living at home: a cross sectional study. *BMC Geriatrics*. 2012;12(1):27.

Croicu C, Chwastiak L, Katon W. Approach to the patient with multiple somatic symptoms. *Med Clin N Am*. 2014;98(5):1070–1095.

Dimsdale JE. Somatic symptom disorders: a new approach in DSM-5. *Die Psychiatrie*. 2103;10:30–32.

Dimsdale JE, Creed F, Escobar, J, Levenson, J. Somatic symptom disorder: an important change in DSM. *J Pscyhosom Res*. 2013;75(3):223–228.

Gierk B, Kohlmann S, Kroenke K, etc. The somatic symptom scale–8 (SSS-8): a brief measure of somatic symptom burden. *JAMA Intern Med*. 2014;174(3):399–407.

Gierk B, Kohlmann S, Toussaint A, Lowe B. Assessing somatic symptom burden. a psychometric comparison of the Patient Health Questionnaire–15 (PHQ-15) and the Somatic Symptom Scale–8 (SSS-8). *J Psychosom Res*. 2015;78(4):352–355.

Grassi, L., Caruso, R., & Nanni, M. G. Somatization and somatic symptom presentation in cancer: a neglected area. *Intern Rev Psychiatry*. 2013;25(1):41–51.

Kleinstauber M, Rief W. Somatoform and related disorders: an update. *Psychiatric Times*. 2015;32(9):1–6.

Kroenke K, Spitzer R, Williams J. The PHQ-15: validity of a new measure for evaluating the severity of somatic symptoms. *Psychosom Med*. 2002;64(2):258–266.

Martin A, Rauh E, Fichter M, Rief W. A one-session treatment for patients suffering from medically unexplained symptoms in primary care: a randomized clinical trial. *Psychosomatics*. 2007;48(4):294–303.

Mundt, A. P. Multiple medication use in somatic symptom disorders: from augmentation to diminution strategies. In: Ritsner M, ed., *Polypharmacy in Psychiatry Practice*. Vol. 1. Dorecht, The Netherlands: Springer; 2013:243–254.

Ravesteign H, Wittkampf K, Lucassen, P, et al. Detecting somatoform disorders in primary care with the PHQ-15. Ann Fam Med. 2009;7(3):232–238.

Shaw RJ, Bernard RS, DeMaso DR. Somatoform disorders. In: Steiner H, ed. *Handbook of Developmental Psychiatry*. London, England: World Scientific; 2011:397–429.

Somashekar B, Jainer A, Wuntakal B. Psychopharmacotherapy of somatic symptoms disorders. *Int Rev Psychiatry*. 2013;25(1):107–115.

Van Dessel N, den Boeft M, van der Wouden JC, et al. Nonpharmacological interventions for somatoform disorders and medically unexplained physical symptoms (MUPS) in adults. *Cochrane Database Syst Rev*. 2014;11(1):CD CD011142. https://doi.org/10.1002/14651858.CD011142.pub2

Weisblatt E, Hindley P, Rask CU. Medically unexplained symptoms in children and adolescents. In: Creed F, Henningsen P, Fink P, eds. *Medically Unexplained Symptoms, Somatisation and Bodily Distress: Developing Better Clinical Services*. New York, NY: Cambridge University Press; 2011:158–174.

12 The Unseen Reality

Sarah is 45-year-old female presenting with a diagnosis of chronic low back and fibromyalgia. However, she was also convinced she had parasites, which she felt crawling on her scalp. She noticed little pods with sticks coming out of them in her feces. She experienced nausea and bloating after meals. She attributed this condition to having lived near a catfish pond. Although undergoing fecal testing by her primary care physician, she had not sought a dermatology, infectious disease, or gastrointestinal consultation reasoning that "they would probably just lose my samples" or "I tried to bring one of the pods in a vial, but it disintegrated before I got to office." Her medication list includes Adderall® and Nuvigil®, secondary to diagnosis of narcolepsy; 140 mg/day of oxycodone; Lyrica®; Zanaflex®; and Voltaren® gel. She had previously been on high doses of methadone, morphine ER, and Nucynta®.

What do you do now?

BACKGROUND

Delusional parasitosis (DP; delusional infestations; aka Ekbom's syndrome) is a psychotic illness, first described in the 17th century, characterized by an unshakable belief of being infested by a parasite, absent supporting medical evidence (Bak et al, 2008,a,b). The estimated incidence is 1.9/100,000, age of onset 55 to 68 years, with females outnumbering males 3:1 (Bailey et al, 2014; Mohammed and Al-Imam, 2016). Average duration is three years but can persist for decades. Morgellons disease is a self-diagnosed, unconfirmed skin condition in which individuals have sores that they believe contain some kind of fibers. Some also experience a sensation of crawling, biting, and stinging on or in their skin (formication). These symptoms can be very painful.

DP beliefs about infestation by insects, worms, mites, lice, fleas, or other organisms may extend to one's home, surroundings, and clothing as being infested (delusional cleptoparasitosis). The description of the manner in which the organism enters via skin or other openings and navigates about is quite vivid. However, general mental abilities are often not compromised (Frean, 2010). In the fifth edition of the *Diagnostic and Statistical Manual of Mental Disorders* (American Psychiatric Association, 2013), DP corresponds with "Delusional Disorder DSM-5 297.1 (F22); Schizophrenia Spectrum and Other Psychotic Disorders."

DP can be primary, secondary, or organic. *Primary DP*, also called monosymptomatic hypochondriacal psychosis, involves a single delusional belief of being infested. *Secondary DP* can occur in the context of other mental disorder like schizophrenia, depression, and dementia. *Organic DP* occurs secondary to organic illness (eg, hypothyroidism, vitamin B12 deficiency, diabetes, cerebrovascular disease, cocaine intoxication, HIV, allergies, and menopausal state). Where parasites do exist, they are believed to be macro-parasites (eg, helminths) or smaller parasites like virus or bacteria. Patients often perceive the parasites as crawling or burrowing into skin.

Discrete bruises, nodular pruritus, ulcers, and scars are frequently produced by patient trying to remove the parasite (self-mutilation). Patients with Morgellons disease commonly seek attention of dermatologist or physicians and may continue seeking different professional/therapies in

Primary/true/autochthonous: Independent of any medical or associated psychiatric condition, there is no additional deterioration of basic mental functioning.

Secondary functional: Associated with psychiatric conditions, such as schizophrenia and depression.

Secondary organic: Caused by medical illness or recreational substance abuse.

Orificial DP: A variant of DP involving body orifices.

Delusory cleptoparasitosis: A form of DP; patients think the organism is in their dwelling.

Delusional infestation: Includes both DP and delusion of infestation with inanimate objects. Patients usually have other psychiatric disorders.

Morgellons disease: Includes delusional infestation with cognitive defects, behavioral changes, tiredness, and other symptoms.

Formication: Similar to DP, but patients are not delusional (ie, they can be convinced with evidence that they do not have a real infestation).

Illusions of parasitosis: Produced by actual physical causes (eg, insulation, static electricity, or fragments that feel like stings and various allergens or materials such as formalin produce dermatitis; such individuals are not delusional and are convinced when the condition is explained.

Adapted from Mohammed M, Al-Imam L, A systematic literature review on delusional parasitosis. *J Dermatol Dermatol Surg.* 2016;20:5–14.

search of a cure. This type of medical odyssey can be expensive and dangerous. Classification and subtypes are shown in Box 12.1.

ASSESSMENT

A number of relevant questions need to be addressed during the assessment of the patient suspected of DP. Could there have been an inflammatory skin response causing itching and dry spots that the patient interprets (somatic hypervigilance and catastrophizing) as parasites? Could there have been a neuropathic component to the sensation of bugs? Are there secondary gain issues?

DP is sometimes difficult to diagnose because many actual skin disorders (eg, allergies, dermatitis, real parasites) can cause the itching sensations. Skin sores or irritation caused by the scratching and use of chemicals may look like other skin disorders. Indeed, the qualitative characteristics (eg, crawling, stinking, prinking etc.) can mimic neuropathic symptoms. As such, DP is often a diagnosis by exclusion. However, the assessment should include a physical examination, skin scrapings, and appropriate lab tests to rule out real infestations and other diseases. Any history of drug use or mental disorders should be investigated. If an infestation has been ruled out, examination by a psychiatrist may be necessary to determine if DP is part of a mental disorder.

Secondary organic DP occurs when a medical illness or substance (medical or recreational) use causes the patient's symptoms. Physical illnesses that can underlie secondary organic DP include hypothyroidism, cancer, cerebrovascular disease, tuberculosis, neurological disorders, vitamin B12 deficiency, and diabetes mellitus. Associated factors in the elderly include senile pruritus, diabetic neuropathy, reduced visual acuity, reduced blood flow, due to arterial stenosis (produces paresthesia), loss of autonomy, depression and low self-esteem, polypharmacy, and frequent taking of over-the-counter drugs, supplements, and herbal remedies.

Structural magnetic resonance images have revealed abnormalities in patients with DP. For example, lesions in the corpus striatum (putamen) and areas of the somatic dorsal striato-thalamo-cortical loop were found in patients with secondary organic DP (Huber et al, 2008). The putamen is known to mediate motor and visuo-tactile perception. Involvement of the striatum along with the noted efficacy of antidopaminergic antipsychotic medication suggests a dopaminergic dysfunction in DP.

Formication can be a trigger for DP, especially the somatically oriented and obsessive-compulsive individual. Medical illnesses associated with formication include menopause (ie, hormone withdrawal), allergies, and drug abuse (eg, cocaine, methamphetamine [amphetamine psychosis]). In the setting of pain, one must rule out opioid toxicity, which can be associated with hallucinations. Environmental factors (airborne irritants) are capable of inducing a crawling sensation in otherwise healthy individuals. However, the patient with PD becomes fixated and obsessed as to its degree and meaning, suffering significant disruption to their quality of life and an inability to carry out their usual social/occupational role.

Examination the skin may well reveal discrete bruises, nodular pruritus, ulcers, and self-mutilation scars resulting from the patient attempting to rid themselves of the parasite. The afflicted patient may produce dust, fibers, scabs, or debris from the skin to support their claim. The specimens are often presented in small container (matchbox, pill container, or a sealed plastic bag; ie, matchbox sign or specimen sign). Indeed, one might find fibers under the skin originating in clothing or the environment. One patient reportedly declared "My creepy crawlies definitely caused anxiety and agitation. I remember fantasizing about cutting my own skin open and ripping my leg muscles to shreds" (Mohammed and Al-Iman, 2016).

There are instances where DP intersects with the law (Shelommi, 2015): (i) competency hearings; (ii) disability claims; (iii) high risk of self-harm during the acute phase of the condition, either from ill-advised forms of self-treatment (such as bathing in bleach or lighting oneself or one's home on fire); and (iv) suicide when treatments fail. Patients with DP may pose a risk to others by viewing pets, family members, or other cohabitants as infested and in need of treatment. Such treatment make take the form of child, elder, or animal abuse or endangerment cases. The intractable nature of DP can lead to paranoia and the belief that the medical community is conspiring against the patient. Cases of harassment, attempted murder, and even one successful murder of doctors by patients unwilling to accept a psychiatric diagnosis have been documented. Malpractice suits, civil cases against pest control companies or landlords for not resolving—or, indeed, for deliberately causing—the infestation have been recorded.

In general, the courts focus on the welfare of persons with DP and those associated with them, especially children. They are sensitive to the patients concerns and acknowledge the physical and psychosocial consequences of DP. The courts have general relied upon the finding of the scientific and medical community, without attempting to confirm the delusion and tend to reject the testimony of those who diagnose the presence of parasites without scientific evidence.

TREATMENT

Building trust and rapport with the patient is an essential, but challenging ingredient to successful treatment. Box 12.2 outlines steps to take to gain the trust of a patient with DP. It is important to help the patient avoid the physician odyssey. This fruitless marry-go-round of repeated assessment and treatment trials can be expensive and dangerous. Supportive psychotherapy and the use of second-generation antipsychotics should be considered as the first line of treatment. The condition is among the most successfully treated delusional disorders, typically through long-term use of atypical antipsychotic medications. However, disease relapse is not uncommon.

Treatment of DP is best coordinated with a dermatologist and psychiatrist. The dermatologist needs to rule out any actual parasites. The person is then referred to a psychiatrist so that their delusion can be treated. Antipsychotic drugs such as risperidone and haloperidol can be very effective. However, people often refuse to accept psychiatric help and, instead, visit many different doctors in a futile search for a treatment that will eradicate the parasites they imagine.

A difficult and important aspect to treatment is convincing the patient that their condition is psychiatric; a trusting doctor–patient is critical.

BOX 12.2 **Some Methods to Gain Trust From a Patient With DP**

- Reassure the patient the condition has been seen before and can be treated.
- Be empathetic and understanding versus dismissive.
- Examine the skin carefully.
- Start nonirritating, local treatment for self-induced injury.
- Attempt to reduce the patient's agitation and preoccupation.
- Offer antidepressant therapy to those patients with depression/anxiety.
- Review the need and potential benefit of joint consultation with other specialists.
- Carry out microbiological/parasitological testing on the patient's specimen(s).

Adapted from Mohammed M, Al-Imam L. A systematic literature review on delusional parasitosis. *J Dermatol Dermatol Surg.* 2016;20:5–14.

Delusions rarely resolve on their own; there is a 50% chance of remission with psychotropic drugs. The clinician needs to be prepared to call upon other specialties. Suicide is a risk. If suspected, the patient should be hospitalized and carefully monitored. In severe DP, the physician may persuade the patient that treatment is necessary because of the psychological impact, telling them that the organism can be virulent in psychologically and physically fragile individuals.

The current first-line drug treatment is risperidone (1–8 mg/day) and olanzapine (5–10 mg/day; atypical or second-generation antipsychotics). Pimozide has been the classical treatment with a recovery rate of 90% but has a high risk for extrapyramidal and cardiac toxicity. Safer first-generation treatments include haloperidol, perphenazine, and sulpiride; metabolic dysfunction is a major risk. Full remission with second-generation antipsychotics in 75% of cases within three months of therapy has been reported.

A depot antipsychotics can be used with the noncompliant patient. Acceptance of a depot may be enhanced by using the hyposensitization motivational strategy (Bahmer and Behmer, 2002). The patient with DP is informed that their condition represents a form of extreme hypersensitivity of the most peripheral skin nerves, not unlike an allergic reaction. Therefore, hyposensitization is needed to return the nerves to normal reactivity. Lepping et al (2015) includes an audio attached that provides an excellent example of how to present the possibility of DP to the patient.

Interestingly, fentanyl citrate, an opiate agonist was associated with an increase in the exaggerated complaints of a patient with DP while naloxone hydrochloride, an opiate antagonist, alleviated DP symptoms. Naloxone also caused euphoria in patients with DP, while the control group reported dysphoria (Botschev and Müller, 1991).

In the case of Sarah, she became vague and gave far-fetched reasons when declining the recommendation that she consult infectious disease specialist, dermatologist, etc. She was not a danger to herself or others, and declined a psychiatric referral. She was more accepting of sleep study referral to better address her narcolepsy but did not follow though. At her three-month follow-up visit, for reasons that are unknown, she did not obtain the recommended the infectious disease consultation but claimed her symptoms had resolved. She just sort of brushed it off (no pun intended).

- Resist the temptation to discount the patient. Get the facts first.
- Consider delusional infestation in patients who present with a fixed belief that they are infested with living or nonliving organisms in the absence of medical evidence.
- Always exclude real infestations first, reviewed by a dermatologist or infectious disease specialist, and obtain appropriate tests.
- Acknowledge the patient's distress without reinforcing false beliefs.
- Most patients require antipsychotic treatment as a means to alleviate symptoms.
- Management ideally requires a multidisciplinary approach, but as patients rarely agree to full psychiatric assessment, physicians who have engaged patients in a trusting relationship should offer medication, if possible with psychiatric advice.
- Doctors, entomologists, and others who commonly see persons with DP should be on alert for patients/clients who indicate that they are treating children or other family members and may want to request a police welfare check if they feel a child is at risk.

Adopted in part form Lepping et al, How to approach delusional infestation. *BMJ*. 2015;350:h1328. https://doi.org/10.1136/bmj.h1328

Further Reading

Bailey CH, Andersen LK, Lowe GC, Pittelkow MR, Bostwick JM, Davis MDP. A population-based study of the incidence of delusional infestation in Olmsted County, Minnesota, 1976–2010. *Br J Dermatol*. 2014;70(5):1130–1135. https://doi.org/10.1111/bjd.12848

Bahmer FA, Bahmer J. Neuroleptic "hyposensitization"—therapy for delusional parasitosis. *Dermatol Psychosomatik*. 2002;3(3):148–149.

Bak R, Tumu P, Hui C, Kay D. A review of delusions of parasitosis, Part 1: Presentation and diagnosis. *Cutis*. 2008a;82(2):123–130.

Bak R, Tumu P, Hui C, Kay D. A review of delusions of parasitosis, Part 2: Treatment options. *Cutis*. 2008b;82:257–264.

Botschev C, Müller N. Opiate receptor antagonists for delusions of parasitosis. *Biol Psychiatry*. 1991;30(5):530–531.

Frean, J. Delusional parasitosis: case series and a review of the literature. *Ann Acad Med Singap*. 2010;11:21–23.

Huber M, Karner M, Kirchler E, Lepping P, Freudenmann RW. Striatal lesions in delusional parasitosis revealed by magnetic resonance imaging. *Prog Neuropsychopharmacol Biol Psychiatry*. 2008;32(8):1967–1971.

Lepping P, Huber M, Freudenmann RW. How to approach delusional infestation *BMJ*. 2015;350:h1328. https://doi.org/10.1136/bmj.h1328

Mohammed M, Al-Imam L. A systematic literature review on delusional parasitosis. *J Dermatol Dermatol Surg*. 2016;20:5–14.

Shelommi M. Delusional infestation/parasitosis and the law: a review. *Psychol Crime Law*. 2015;21(8):747–763. https://doi.org/10.1080/1068316X.2015.1038265

13 There Are Not Enough Sheep

Natalie has been in pain management for seven years. Over time she has developed problems sleeping, which she had not had in the past. She has some problems with sleep onset but also awakens early. Morning is one of her worse times of the day regarding pain. She has tried a number of over-the-counter sleep aids. She currently takes a tranquilizer and a sedative-hypnotic at night with some, but limited, help. Her worsening pain leads her to believe she has a new or progressive injury.

What do you do now?

BACKGROUND

There are a variety of sleep disorders including insomnia, restless leg syndrome, sleep apnea, parasomnias. Insomnia and sleep apnea are the ones most associated with chronic pain. Insomnia is characterized by difficulty with sleep onset, frequent awakening, early morning awakening, and nonrestorative sleep. Sleep-onset latency correlates with hyperarousal (cognitive and somatic), is independent of depression and pain intensity, and often becomes a conditioned phenomenon. Sleep apnea is characterized by pauses in breathing during sleep, causing the body take in less oxygen and frequent arousal.

Sleep disturbance impairs cognitive/physical functioning, quality of life, and occupational performance. It can affect pain threshold, pain modulation, pain perception, and hyperalgesia (Artner et al, 2013; Haack et al, 2020). Sleep impairment is a more reliable predictor of daytime pain intensity than pain intensity is of sleep impairment. Sleep impairment is also more strongly associated with depression than pain severity or opioid use. Sleep medications have no impact of pain severity or depression. Insomnia affects 9% to 15% general population but up to 88% of patients with chronic pain. Artner et al (2013) reported 42% of patients with sleep deprivation (<4 hour/night) due to pain were talking analgesics.

Poor sleep is not only associated with chronic pain but also can contribute to the development and maintenance of chronic pain. For example, Sanders et al (2016) found poor sleep quality predicted the onset of painful temporomandibular disorder, and Miranda et al (2013), in low back pain. Thus, insomnia significantly increases the risk of developing chronic pain disorders in previously pain-free individuals. Bonvanie et al (2016) reported that 38% of emerging adults (18–25 years old) with severe sleep problems at initial evaluation had chronic pain at a three-year follow-up, compared with 14% of those without initial sleep problems. The relationship between sleep and pain was stronger in women.

A 2013 review concluded:

The most salient findings are that both sleep disturbance and pain tend to increase with age; African Americans exhibit worse objective and subjective sleep impairments and greater clinical and experimental pain sensitivity than Caucasians; and females exhibit worse

> **BOX 13.1   Possible Mechanisms by Which Sleep Disorders Affect Pain**
>
> - Dysregulate the endogenous opioid system and attenuates the analgesic efficacy of mu opioid receptor agonists.
> - Abolishes the monoamine potential of opioidergic antinociception.
> - Alters mu and delta opioid receptor function in mesolimbic circuits.
> - Diminishes basal endogenous opioid levels.
> - Downregulates central opioid receptors.
> - Associated with elevated cytokines, especially interleukin 6.
> - Associated with increased in opioid consumption.

objective and subjective sleep impairments and greater clinical and experimental pain sensitivity than males. (Finan et al, 2013, p. 1548)

Box 13.1 outlines some of the proposed mechanisms by which sleep affects pain and the impact of opioids as summarized by Finn et al (2013).

ASSESSMENT

A detailed medical examination and history including assessment of psychiatric and substance-related factors, risk factors for other sleeping disorders (sleep apnea), obesity, diabetes, increased neck circumference, and upper airway anatomical changes should be conducted. An analysis of the patient's sleep pattern (eg, difficulty falling asleep vs awakenings vs poor sleep), frequency and duration of insomnia, identification of nocturnal symptoms, impact on daytime activities and functioning, and any past or current treatments and responses will help to clarify the problem. For example, patients can be awakened by an end-of-dose phenomenon. They can experience a type of miniature withdrawal. This is most evident if their pain is worse when they first awake or if they find themselves taking medicine in the middle of the night.

Examining nighttime routines; caffeine intake; napping during the day; headaches; awakening due to other medical problems such as pain, urination, or muscle spasms; shift work; and stress may identify some therapeutic targets. When possible, the patient should complete a two-week sleep diary and a sleep questionnaire such as the Insomnia Severity Index (Morin et al, 2011), a short 7-item rating the patients' perceptions of their insomnia.

A referral to sleep clinic may be needed. It is critical to rule out sleep apnea. The three common types are (i) obstructive, (ii) central, and (iii) mixed sleep apnea. Obstructive sleep apnea (OSA) is caused by a partial or complete blockage of the airways during sleep. Central sleep apnea (CSA) is often related to medical problems and conditions affecting the brain stem. Mixed sleep apnea is a combination of both OSA and CSA symptoms. There is strong evidence of a close relationship between opioids and sleep breathing disorders, particularly CSA. This appears especially true for methadone, high opioid dosing (>200 mg morphine equivilant dose [MED]), and combining opioids with benzodiazepines (Cheatle and Webster, 2015). One study (Correa et al, 2015) reported the prevalence of CSA in chronic opioid users at 24%. However, other estimates range as high as 90% (Panagiotou et al, 2012). Both chronic use of opioids and OSA have been associated with hypogonadism in men. Attempts to use replacement therapy for those on opioids will likely be compromised in the presence of uncorrected OSA. Indeed, in the absence of sleep study one could erroneously conclude that the hypogonadism is secondary to opioids.

TREATMENT: MEDICATIONS

Sedative-hypnotics. In general, medications should be used for the short-term to break of fatigue and insomnia. Traditional sedative-hypnotics (Ambien®, Sonata®, and Lunesta®) are approved for 30-day use. Belsomra® (suvorexant) and the recently approved Dayvigo® (lemborexant) are considered a sedative-hypnotic. However, they are believed to be an antagonist of orexin receptors. The orexin neuropeptide signaling system is a central promoter of wakefulness. Thus, they differ from other sedative-hypnotics and benzodiazepines.

Benzodiazepines. Benzodiazepines (eg, alprazolam [Xanax®], lorazepam [Ativan®], diazepam [Valium®], clonazepam [Klonopin®]) should be use with caution. A short- or intermediate-acting benzodiazepine receptor agonists (eg, zaleplon [Sonata®], zolpidem [Ambien®], eszopiclone [Lunesta®], triazolam [Halcion®], or temazepam Restroil®]) are commonly used. Benzodiazepines have sedative, anxiolytic, muscle relaxant, and anticonvulsant properties secondary to their effect on the γ-aminobutyric acid receptor.

Newer nonbenzodiazepine sedative-hypnotics, such as zaleplon and ramelteon (Rozerem®) possess only sedative properties. They can reduce sleep latency but are not effective in reducing wakefulness after sleep onset. Intermediate-acting agents such as temazepam and eszopiclone can be used to improve sleep maintenance. Acute insomnia can be treated for two to four weeks. Chronic insomnia should be treated intermittently (eg, 2–5 nights/week). Eszopiclone and zolpidem have been studied for up to 12 months. Patients receiving long-term sedative-hypnotics should be followed and re-evaluated at least as often as every six months.

Benzodiazepine-related side effects include anterograde amnesia and rebound insomnia when discontinued. Tolerance to benzodiazepines can develop after one month of use. These agents can be particularly dangerous in elderly patients because of the increased risk for falling. Nonbenzodiazepine sedative-hypnotic agents have demonstrated similar efficacy to benzodiazepines but have the advantage of less residual sedation.

Benzodiazepines should not be used in conjunction with opioids secondary to sedation, confusion, and possible overdose (Rajput et al, 1999). One study reported that 301 of 498 (60.4%) patients who died while on opioid therapy and whose death was judged to be related to the opioid were also taking benzodiazepines. Patients who take opioids should avoid taking benzodiazepines, barbiturates, or alcohol before going to sleep, and physicians should be extremely cautious about prescribing benzodiazepines and barbiturates for sleep or any other reason to patients who are on opioids (Gomes et al, 2011).

Antidepressants. Patients with comorbid depression may be candidates for low-dose sedating antidepressant therapy (eg, trazodone [Desyrel®], mirtazapine [Remeron®], doxepin [Silenor®], and amitriptyline [Elavil®]). In addition, to improving sleep and mood, antidepressants can have analgesic effects. However, tricyclic antidepressants, such as amitriptyline and doxepin, have been associated with anticholinergic effects (eg, urinary retention, constipation, dry mouth) and cardiac conduction abnormalities. Daytime sedation can also occur. Trazodone does not produce these anticholinergic effects but has been associated with orthostatic hypotension and priapism in men. Dependence is rare. Therefore, trazodone may be especially useful for patients with a history of substance abuse. When used in combination with other serotonin-based drugs, it is important to be aware of the possibility of serotonin surge syndrome.

Over the counter. Sedating antihistamines may be useful in the short term for mild insomnia. However, they can alter sleep architecture and have anticholinergic side effects. Caution should be exercised when using with the elderly because of an increased risk of falling. Dietary supplements (eg, valerian, melatonin, and l-tryptophan) have been useful. In general, melatonin at 3 mg has only been found useful in sleep–wake cycle disorders. One can also consider the melatonin receptor agonist ramelteon. Valerian root is a minor tranquilizer and hypnotic used at 400 to 900 mg per night. These substances are not regulated by the US Food and Drug Administration. Therefore, content labeling may not be accurate.

Cannabinoids. Preliminary research into cannabis and insomnia suggests that cannabidiol may have therapeutic potential for the treatment of insomnia. Delta-9 tetrahydrocannabinol may decrease sleep latency but could impair sleep quality long term. Studies investigating cannabinoids and OSA suggest that synthetic cannabinoids such as nabilone (Casemet®) and dronabinol (Marinol®) may have short-term benefit for sleep apnea due to their modulatory effects on serotonin-mediated apneas. Cannabidiol may hold promise for rapid eye movement sleep behavior disorder and excessive daytime sleepiness, while nabilone may reduce nightmares associated with posttraumatic stress disorder and may improve sleep among patients with chronic pain.

Behavioral. Behavioral approaches include a variety of strategies. *Stimulus control* refers to the sleep environment. The bed and bedroom should be reserved for sleeping. Watching television, browsing the iPad, eating, reading, talking, phone conversations, etc. should be done elsewhere. If not asleep in 20 minutes or so, one should leave the bed and return when tired. The bedtime worrier should set aside a "worry time," if needed, before going to bed. The body becomes classically conditioned to associate the bedroom and sleeping with worry. Daytime problems can manifest themselves at night. The brain no longer associates the bedroom with only sleeping but as a time to mull-over problems.

Sleep hygiene refers to habits that interfere with sleep; caffeine and nicotine are the most common. Both are stimulants. Caffeine should be eliminated after 12 o'clock noon. The impact of smoking can be determined by how often the patient awakens to have a cigarette. Alcohol can result in drowsiness but is associated with fragmented sleep. It is best to avoid naps. Increasing exercise and physical activity can help.

Cognitive-behavioral therapy (CBT) has been used in combination with the previously described behavioral interventions. CBT helps patients alter their beliefs and unrealistic expectations about sleep. Meta-analysis comparing CBT (stimulus control, sleep restriction therapy, relaxation therapy, cognitive therapy, sleep hygiene education; 6–8 sessions) versus hypnotics showed similar short term outcomes but "all these studies showed that at 10–24 months CBT alone, but not CBT plus hypnotic, continued to show improvement" (Silber, 2005, p. 803). This suggests that sedative-hypnotics may interfere with the integration of CBT or that the patient focused more the medication than the therapy. Table 13.1 lists a number of dos and don'ts recommended by Tanzi et al (2011).

TABLE 13.1 **Dos and Don'ts**

Do	Don't
Establish a predictable sleep/wake schedule	Use stimulants for up to six hours before bedtime
Have a winding down period before bedtime	Use alcohol before bedtime
Use the bedroom only for sleep and sex	Use medications that can disrupt sleep
Create a sleep-friendly environment: quiet, cool, and dark	Have a heavy meal within three hours of bedtime
Limit naps to one hour or less	Take naps after 3 pm
	Lay in bed awake and fighting to go to sleep
	Exercise within three hours of bedtime
	Have caffeine after 12 noon

- Sleep impairments (i) are a more reliable predictor of pain than pain is of sleep impairment and (ii) contribute to the development and maintenance of chronic pain, and (iii) are predicted more by depression than by pain severity or opioid use.
- Sleep medications do not impact of pain severity or depression.
- Sleep medication use is highly correlated with poor sleep quality, duration, and efficiency.
- The use of nighttime medications is not likely to overcome poor sleep hygiene.

Further Reading

Artner J, Cakir B, Spiekermann JA, et al. Prevalence of sleep deprivation in patients with chronic neck and back pain: a retrospective evaluation of 1016 patients. *J Pain Res.* 2013:6;1–6.

Bonvanie I, Oldehinkel A, Rosmalen J, Janssens K. Sleep problems and pain: a longitudinal cohort study in emerging adults. *Pain.* 2016;157(4):957–963.

Chapman JB, Lehman CL, Elliott J, Clark J. Sleep quality and the role of sleep medications for veterans with chronic pain. *Pain Med.* 2006;7(2):105–114.

Cheatle MD, Webster LR. Opioid therapy and sleep disorders: risks and mitigation strategies. *Pain Med.* 2015;6(Suppl): S22–S26.

Correa D, Farney RJ, Chung F, Prasad A, Lam D, Wong J. Chronic opioid use and central sleep apnea: a review of the prevalence, mechanisms, and perioperative considerations. *Anesth Analg.* 2015;120:1273–1285.

Finan PH, Goodin B, Smith MT. The association of sleep and pain: an update and a path forward. *J Pain.* 2013;14(12):1539–1552.

Gomes T, Mamdani MM, Dhalla IA, Paterson JM, Juurlink DN. Opioid dose and drug-related mortality in patients with nonmalignant pain. *Arch Intern Med.* 2011;171:686–691.

Haack M, Simpson N, Sethna N, Kaur S, Mullington J. Sleep deficiency and chronic pain: potential underlying mechanisms and clinical implications. *Neuropsychopharmacology.* 2020;45(1):205–216. https://doi.org/10.1038/s41386-019-0439-z

Miranda H, Viikari-Juntura E, Punnett L, Riihimaki H. Occupational loading, health behavior and sleep disturbance as predictors of low-back pain. *Scand J Work Environ Health.* 2008;34(6):411–419.

Morin CM, Belleville G, Bélanger L, Ivers H. The insomnia severity index: psychometric indicators to detect insomnia cases and evaluate treatment response. *Sleep*. 2011;34(5):601–608.

Oliver RL, Taylor A, Oliver R. Chronic insomnia and pain under-reported and under-treated, chronic insomnia coexists with—and perpetuates—chronic pain. *Pract Pain Manage*. 2002;2(6):1–4.

Panagiotou I, Mystakidou K. Non-analgesic effects of opioids: opioids' effects on sleep (including sleep apnea). *Curr Pharm Des*. 2012;18:6025–6033.

Rajput V, Bromley S. Chronic insomnia: A practical review. *Am Fam Physician*. 1999;60:1431–1437.

Sanders AE, Akinkugbe AA, Bair E, et al. Subjective sleep quality deteriorates before development of painful temporomandibular disorder. *J Pain*. 2016;17(6):669–677.

Schutte-Rodin S, Broch L, Buysse D, Dorsey C, Sateia M. Clinical guideline for the evaluation and management of chronic insomnia in adults. *J Clin Sleep Med*. 2008;4(5):487–504.

Silber MH. Chronic insomnia. *NEJM*. 2005;353(8):803–810.

Tanzi M, Lodolce AE, Prasad B. Management of insomnia: considerations for patients with chronic pain. Pract Pain Manage. 2011;11(10):48–62.

Wittert G The relationship between sleep disorders and testosterone. Curr Opin Endocrinol Diabetes Obes. 2014;21(3):239–243.

14 The Easy but Harmful Solution

Helen is 49-year-year female with a history
of back, leg, arm, and neck pain; status post
low-back surgery; multilevel spondylotic changes
in her low back and neck; fibromyalgia; anxiety;
panic disorder; chronic obstructive pulmonary
disease; nicotine and caffeine overuse; migraine
headache; and a very reactive personality.
Her current milligram morphine equivalent
approximates 120/day. Her chronic widespread
pain rating is 7/10, and she states that it is worse
compared to the last visit. She is on several
medication from outside your clinic including
Klonopin®, Cymbalta®, and Zyprexa®. Her
husband controls her medications to minimize
any overuse. She denies the use of illicit drugs
or alcohol. Some recent family issues appear to
be aggravating her pain. She insists on the need
to increase her pain medicine and an OK to have
her other doctor increase her Klonopin®.

What do you do now?

BACKGROUND

America appears to have emerged as a medication-oriented country. We use more than our fair share of psychotropic medications, alprazolam being the most frequently prescribed (Miller, 2016), and opioids (https://www.incb.org/documents/Publications/AnnualReports/AR2015/English/AR_2015_E.pdf. Accessed November, 2020). Nearly 17% of American adults used one or more psychiatric drugs in 2013, up from 10% in 2011. We search for the most immediate and least time-consuming solution. The hope for a quick fix, or at least a brief escape or respite from symptoms, outweighs concerns over long-term consequences. Children are being parented by electronics and come into adulthood ill-equipped to effectively manage the inevitable stresses and disappointments of life. An increasing demand for, and promise of, being taken care of has replaced the once rugged individualism." There is a reason the United States is a prime target for drug dealers exporting illicit drugs.

The concepts of *salience* and *resilience* have taken on importance in the chronic pain literature. Simply put, *salience* (Borsook et al, 2013) is the amount of attention, meaning, and importance one gives to pain. *Resilience* (Sturgeon and Zautra, 2010) is an ability to withstand unpleasantries. Genetics and functional brain imaging has suggested that some individuals are wired to be more aware and physiologically sensitive than others (James, 2013; Wager et al, 2013). However, epigenetics has taught us that we can influence the expression of these tendencies (Descalzi et al, 2015). If the words uttered by a person in a white lab coat can impact the effect of an inert substance on the experience of pain (Benedetti et al, 2011), it stands to reason that self-talk could also be influential.

Advertising specialists have known and capitalized on this notion for decades. Nearly 70% of direct to consumer television marketing is by pharmaceutical companies, and it is tax deductible. A brief search on the internet ("Medications for Chronic Pain," n.d.) uncovered a list of no less than 67 medications for chronic pain; all but three were opioid-based. Direct-to-consumer advertising seems to be able to transform a variety of medications into life-altering, life-enhancing, if not life-saving, products. The adverse events are often minimized. Indeed, about 40% of violations in drug ads cited by the US Food and Drug Administration (FDA) between 2004 and 2013 relate to risk minimization ("Do TV DTC Ads," 2014).

Commercials tend to medicalize the problems, making them more palatable. Unfortunately, this also encourages placing the burden of cure of the medical clinician. How often is the viewer encouraged to "discuss this with your physician"? When did you last hear a commercial tell a patient suffering from headache to get some stress management, relaxation therapy, increase exercise, improve nutrition, decrease caffeine, and discontinue smoking. To be fair, there may be a need for effective medication(s) and appropriate prescribing. Companies do need profits to reinvest in research and development. But the pendulum seems to have swung too far.

We all want to look and feel better, whatever that may mean, with the least effort. We seem to be society less concerned about our own healthcare than other aspects of life, (eg, appearance). Witness the dramatic increase in plastic surgery of almost every type, even among teenagers. In place of a car, contribution to a college fund, vacation trip, etc. teenage girls are getting breast augmentation and other forms of plastic surgery—64,000 in 2013 alone. One wonders if it is more for the child or the parent (vicarious living). The human brain does not reach a level of maturity to make and understand the implications of such a decision until at least 20 years of age.

By virtue of the media, past history, and the report of friends, patients have come to expect they will leave the physician's office with one or more prescriptions. This seems true for benzodiazepines as indicated by an increase of 67% in the number of persons filling a prescription for a benzodiazepine between 1996 and 2013. Not only are patients angry if they do not get a prescription, but they feel dismissed by the clinician. Although the prescribing of opioids has been on the decline as of 2012, there has been an increase in benzodiazepine prescribing. Furthermore, despite the fact that the co-utilization of benzodiazepines with opioids increases the risk of overdose death by nearly fourfold, the rate of co-prescribing almost doubled from 2001 and 2013, with the death rate involving benzodiazepines increasing some sevenfold from 1999 and 2015 (National Institute on Drug Abuse, 2020). This fact prompted the FDA to initiate a black-box warning for the co-utilization of benzodiazepines with opioids.

ASSESSMENT

Although "chemical coping" is not an official diagnosis, it is descriptive of many patients with chronic pain. The definition of pain necessitates the involvement of emotional (psychological) factors (ie, "Pain is a sensory and emotional experience"). Medical/pharmacological intervention has become the dominate approach to physical and mental illness/disease. In some instances, this is the best and only option. There appears to be a lot of lip service paid to more behavioral/psychological and alternative approaches but little in the way of critical support (insurance coverage) and education. Indeed, children learn early on about getting regular, sometimes excessive, medical intervention as indicated the concern over the use of antibiotics; which has significantly decreased as of about 2000. On the other hand, physicians are having to confront new and stronger illness-causing strains.

Chemical copers (CCs) manifest a number of different features. They are psychologically, and often physiologically, dependent on medication(s). They defer responsibility for anything that happens in their life and take a position of hopelessness and helplessness. While they may accept that psychological factors can be influencing their symptoms, they interpret the symptoms as physiological in nature and requiring medical intervention. Everything in their world is overpowering. Their perceived lack of control impugns a sense of meaninglessness to self-oriented therapy (eg, behavior/psychological therapy, exercise, diet, etc.). They may improve with medication increases, but it is time-limited.

CCs will beg, cajole, barging, plead, and even make threats. At times they will involve a support person to help make their case. CCs will engage others in the waiting room in conversation as a means of gathering information. They will cite other patients who they feel have been given preferential treatment, without knowing the facts. They tend to come at the most inopportune time. They come prepared, and do not hesitate, to debate the issue. They will appeal to the clinician's humanity. They will insist on an explanation as a means of placing the clinician on the defensive; no explanation will suffice. Psychological testing is likely to reveal a mixture of somatic preoccupation, dependency, manipulation, anxiety, and high levels emotional reactivity. However, CCs often declare themselves by their behavior pattern. No doubt many are actually distressed, but medicating them further is often not a good strategy.

TREATMENT

As recently as 2019, Kirsch noted,

> Antidepressants are supposed to work by fixing a chemical imbalance, specifically, a lack of serotonin or norepinephrine in the brain. However, analyses of the published and the unpublished clinical trial data are consistent in showing that most (if not all) of the benefits of antidepressants in the treatment of depression and anxiety are due to the placebo response, and the difference in improvement between drug and placebo is not clinically meaningful. . . . Other treatments (e.g., psychotherapy and physical exercise) produce the same benefits as antidepressants and do so without the side effects and health risks of the active drugs. Psychotherapy and placebo treatments also show a lower relapse rate than that reported for antidepressant medication. (Kirsch, 2019, p. 1)

Likewise, Dr. Allen Frances, chair of the DSM IV Task Force, explains "We have more deaths in emergency rooms now from prescribed psychiatric medication than we do for street drugs" (quoted in Ericson, 2014). And, as broadly applied diagnoses will have psychiatrists, and primary care providers, prescribe these pills to younger and younger patients, hospitals across the country may soon face a patient generation that has come to think of the pains of everyday life as treatable illnesses. If pills are needed to fix all ills, is there any such thing as a healthy mind (ie, one capable of adapting and solving problems)?

In the ideal situation, the patient would be referred, and would participate, in the therapy appropriate to their needs (eg, cognitive therapy, biofeedback, relaxation/meditation, stress management, dietary counseling, family therapy, exercise, etc.). However, CCs will have a plethora of excuses. The clinician must guard themselves against being ensnared. "Oh, come on doc, just this once!"; "You have no idea what it has been like lately. I just need something for the short run"; "If you could be in my shoes for just a day, you would understand." There are also the veiled threats: "Don't blame me if I run out early"; "No wonder some people go to the street or friends for help"; "If you want me to stop drinking, give me something that helps the pain."

There is no easy answer. It is paramount that the clinician's psychological sophistication, insight, and skills outweigh that of the patient. Remaining clam, firm, and sympathetic is essential. "Trust me, I understand what you are going through. Over the years I have seen it many times. Increasing medications will not solve the problem, and may make things worse". You must also be cautious about trying to make a suitable substitution such hydroxyzine or buspirone (BuSpar®) in place of a benzodiazepine for anxiety/stress. The behavior exists because it has been reinforced in the past. If you succumb to their request, you will reinforce this medication-seeking behavior, rendering it more recalcitrant. Ignoring it will probably bring about what the behavioral experts call an extinction burst. That is, the patient will become emotional and the requests will escalate, for a while, at least. Some may have a tantrum—yell, cry, curse, stomp out, slam doors, etc. It is CCs' behavior that one is trying to address and not necessarily a particular drug.

One should briefly review lifestyle habits and behaviors that could be contributing such as excessive caffeine, catastrophizing, poor pacing, expectation, deconditioning, etc. It may appear to fall on deaf ears, but this is our job, and it needs to be documented in the encounter note. You should keep a supply of hand-outs, booklets, instructional material, and referral information available. Taking a few minutes to assess barriers that patients believe to be preventing them from engaging in what they know will be beneficial (motivational interviewing; see Section II of this volume) can help to redirect the narrative back to the patient. In some instances, simply giving one or two quick tips and agreeing to see the patients back sooner than usual to check on their progress can assuage the situation.

KEY POINTS TO REMEMBER

- Yielding to the patient's request for additional medication to cope reinforces chemical coping behavior.
- Life is not a chemical deficiency.
- Pain is not an opioid deficiency.
- Began instructing and encouraging the use of self-help strategies early in the treatment process.

- "Give a man a fish, and you feed him for a day. Teach a man to fish, and you feed him for a life time" (Old Chinese proverb).
- Remain vigilant regarding the co-utilization of benzodiazepines and opioids.
- Be the clinician you patient needs, not just the one they want.

Further Reading

Benedetti F, Carlino E, Pollo A. How placebos change the patient's brain. *Neuropsychopharmacology*. 2011;36(1):339–354.

Borsook D, Edwards R, Elman I, Becerra L, Levine J. Pain and analgesia: the value of salience circuits. *Prog Neurobiol*. 2013;104:93–105.

Descalzi G, Ikegami D, Ushijima T, Nestler E, Zachariou V, Narita M. Epigenetic mechanisms of chronic pain. *Trends Neurosci*. 2015;38(4):237–246.

Do TV DTC ads overstate Rx drug risks? FDA may make changes that put patients at risk. *Pharma Marketing Blog*. http://pharmamkting.blogspot.com/2014/02/do-tv-dtc-ads-overstate-rx-drug-risks.html. Published February 18, 2014. Accessed June 22, 2019.

Ericson J. Pill for every ill. *Newsweek*. https://www.newsweek.com/2014/02/07/pill-every-ill-245476.html. Published February 6, 2014.

Frances, AJ. *Saving Normal: An Insider's Revolt Against Out-of-Control Psychiatric Diagnosis, DSM-5, Big Pharma, and the Medicalization of Ordinary Life*. New York, NY: William Morrow; 2013.

Kirsch I. Placebo effect in the treatment of depression and anxiety. *Front Psychiatr*. 2019;10:128–134.

James S. Human pain and genetics: some basics. *Brit J Pain*. 2013;7(4):171–178.

Medications for chronic pain. *Drugs.com*. http://www.drugs.com/condition/chronic-pain.html. Accessed June 17, 2019.

Miller SG. 1 in 6 Americans takes a psychiatric drug. Sci Am. https://www.scientificamerican.com/article/1-in-6-americans-takes-a-psychiatric-drug/. Published December 13, 2016. Accessed June, 2020.

National Institute on Drug Abuse. Overdose death rates. http://www.drugabuse.gov/related-topics/trends-statistics/overdose-death-rates. Published May 2020. Accessed July 2020.

Sturgeon JA, Zautra AJ. Resilience: a new paradigm for adaptation to chronic pain. *Curr Pain Headache Rep*. 2010;14:105–112.

Wager TD, Atlas, LY, Lindquist MA, Roy M, Woo CW, Kross E. An fMRI-based neurologic signature of physical pain. *N Engl J Med*. 2013;368:1388–1397.

15 Is This All There Is?

Life is a tale . . . full of sound and fury, signifying nothing.
—William Shakespeare (Macbeth, Act 5, Scene 5)

Martha has had chronic pain for over 10 years. She has been to several doctors and clinics before coming to you. She has been through all types of procedures and medicines. She has been in your clinic for about one year. She always seems irritable and unhappy. Her pain complaints have always been somewhat nonspecific. She insists that her pain and life are no better on the medication you are prescribing. Although she is already at a higher-than-average dose, she demands that you increase it. When refused, she angrily accuses you of not wanting to help her and insists that you "must do something" to reduce her pain.

What do you do now?

BACKGROUND

Anger is a complex emotional (Spielberger, 1988). State anger (SA) refers to a transitory emotional-physiological condition consisting of subjective feelings and physiological activation (arousal). SA occurs in response to a specific, and present, situation. It can vary in intensity and fluctuates over short periods of time. Trait anger is a stable personality dimension characterized by a predisposition or proneness to experience SA. Some patients will express anger directly and overtly (ie, anger-out); others will suppress it or become passive-aggressive and indirect (ie, anger-in). Trait anger-out is defined by the dispositional tendency to regulate anger through direct verbal or physical expression. This may include verbal insults or aggression, sarcasm, arguing, physical expressions (eg, striking out, slamming doors, etc.), or what is commonly referred to as losing one's temper.

There are at least three cognitive aspects to anger (Trost et al, 2012): goal frustration, external attributions (ie, blame), and perceived injustice. Patients with chronic pain often become frustrated with their inability to participate in valued, self-enhancing, and reinforcing activities. Anger is often generated by the assigning of blame (attribution).The target of the patients' anger may include medical and mental health providers, the legal system, third-party payer, employers, significant others, God, self, or even the whole world (Fernandez and Wasan, 2009; Okifuji et al, 1999). Patients with chronic pain often perceive themselves as victims of injustice. Their thoughts center on attributions of blame, the magnitude of loss, and irreparability of loss (Sullivan et al, 2008).

Trait anger-out appears to have the effect of increasing pain sensitivity in the experimental setting (see Bruehl et al, 2009). Neuroimaging data reveal the presence of overlapping neuro circuits for pain and anger, especially in the limbic system. A dysfunctional endogenous opioid system has been proposed as a mechanism regulating the activity among the different cortical regions. Inadequate endogenous opioid inhibitory activity is hypothesized to be responsible for the link between trait anger-out and pain. In addition, negative emotion (ie, anger) has been associated with increased level of proinflammatory substance such as interleukin 6 (Miyamoto et al, 2013). These proinflammatory substances have been associated with the development and maintenance of pathological pain (Zhou et al, 2016).

In general, elevated trait anger-out, in the absence of direct expression, is associated with increased pain sensitivity. However, for individuals with high trait anger-out tendencies, behavioral expression of anger can result in diminished pain. That is, anger expression triggers an endogenous opioid inhibitory system, which is otherwise relatively inactive. Thus, for individuals with a predominately anger-out style, expressing their anger may be functional and adaptive. Deliberate attempts to suppress anger by subjects with elevated anger-out scores have been associated with even greater pain responsiveness (Burns et al, 2007). The direct expression of anger in those with high trait anger dispositions may reduce pain sensitivity, at least in the short term, and thus be reinforcing to the patient.

Opioids have been found to be effective in controlling agitation (Brown et al, 2010; Husebo et al, 2014) and impulsiveness (Love et al, 2009). Their presence may help to modulate this dysfunctional system. However, the reduction or discontinuation of opioids may be associated with a rebound effect and could be part of what Manhapra et al (2018) describe a protracted abstinence syndrome, which includes an element of agitation.

The rate at which patients express dissatisfaction with their pain management ranges from 15% to as much as 42%, depending on the treatment and pain diagnosis—27% for diabetic neuropathy and 42% for peripheral neuropathy (Parkoohi et al, 2015). Several factors are related to patient frustration and dissatisfaction including limited options, finances, distance of care, insurance carrier, degree of invasiveness, absence of a quick fix, and painful effects of increasing activity (a common goal of pain management). Furthermore, satisfaction with care does not always correlate with satisfaction with outcome. Both appear to be related to compliance. Not all dissatisfied patients become angry and act out, but some do.

The behaviors displayed by the angry and dissatisfied patient vary in kind and intensity (Box 15.1). At times, these behavior can become quite egregious and disruptive. There are at least four groups of patients that may display the kind of behavior described in our case study: (i) drug abusers, (ii) personality disordered, (iii) mood disordered, and (iv) the well-control legitimate patients. The drug abuser may be diverting a significant portion of the prescription either for financial gain or to acquire a more desirable illicit drug. A reduction in the dose or change to a drug with a lower street

BOX 15.1   **Characteristics of the Difficult Patient**

- Unrealistic expectations of cure
- Difficult to communicate with
- Vague and shifting complaints
- Undue concerns (eg, about minor symptoms)
- Invoke feelings like anger, frustration, anxiety, dread, and guilt
- Rambling, unfocused: "Everything hurts"
- Raises new problems as visit ends: "Oh, by the way . . ."
- Make inappropriate demands/requests (eg, additional pain medicine, increased phone contact or clinic appointments, etc.)
- Manipulative, hostile, exploitative, rude, demanding, dissatisfied, controlling, lying, litigious
- "Boundary busting": seductive (sexually or otherwise), dependent, clinging
- Resistant to health professionals' recommendations: underappreciative
- Poor adherence with treatment: inconsistent drug use, missed appointments
- Excessive preoccupation with physical disease

value could prompt a reaction. This is sometimes hard to detect but the use of random drug screens and/or pill counts may help. Often such individuals are clever enough to take a sufficient amount of their drug to ensure that it is present on a routine drug screen.

Such patients may threaten legal action. The likelihood of a patient initiating legal action is increased by (i) a factor of 3 if they feel coerced, (ii) a factor of 3.5 if experienced anger from and/or for the clinician, and (iii) factor of 3.5 if they felt the physician was financially motivated. The likelihood of a patient initiating legal action is 78% less for those indicting that they trusted their doctor (Fishbain et al, 2008).

Patient satisfaction appears to relate more to the relationship between expectations and the clinical outcome than the outcome itself (Hirsh et al, 2005). The patient's perception of the clinician's effort and involvement also appears more important than the actual clinical outcome. Carlson et al (2003) found the level and type of communication to be critical factors. Indeed, Comley and DeMeyer (2001) noted that over 90% of patients reported being satisfied with their pain management despite significant levels of pain and an ineffective treatment suggesting the involvement of other psychological factors.

Empathy has been defined as "the capacity to recognize emotions experienced by another." Several types of empathy have been identified, including cognitive, emotional, trait, and state empathy (Newton, 2013). Imaging studies have uncovered different neurosignatures for affective-perceptual and cognitive-evaluative empathy (Fan et al, 2011). Longitudinal and cross-sectional studies (Hojat et al, 2009; Newton et al, 2008; Neumann et al, 2011) have revealed a significant decline in empathy during the third year of medical school and extending into residency. The burden of patient care, practice economics, changing regulations, and a poorly balance personal life can leave any clinician vulnerable. Being aware of what type of patient can push your buttons and self-monitoring your response can save time, embarrassment, and wasted emotional resources. At times, it can be difficult to find the proper balance between empathy and indifference. Emotional control is an important commodity in the context of discussion making. The clinician is held to fairly high standard when it comes to interacting with patients.

ASSESSMENT

Careful monitoring of the patient, behavioral observational, and random checks can be revealing. At times, the patient's expression of anger is a veiled attempt to cover-up aberrant drug behavior. There may be intentional diversion within the family. The index of suspicion for this should be increased in the case of family member(s) attending the clinic meeting with the patient, especially where the patient is elderly, seems compromised physically and cognitively, and wherein the bulk of the information is provided by the significant other. Situations where the family is financially disadvantaged and wherein apparently healthy individuals are unemployed should also create a concern.

Embedded in this group of the angry and dissatisfied patient is the pseudo-intellect and disease-convicted patient. These terms are descriptive and not intended to be degrading. The pseudointellectual patient often makes awkward attempts at the use of medical jargon. Statement such as "The pain goes down my soriatic nerve" and "I have bulging discices up and down my spine" are common. They often embellish the severity of their problem: "My doctor does not know how I am even walking"; "My problems are so bad that not even surgery will help (if fact, there is no surgical problem)"; "Any minor accident could put me in a wheelchair"; or "My conditioned has worsened to the point where I sometimes need help to bath or shower and dress." These statements are often made despite appearing quite functional in the office and absent any supporting data. Admittedly, these exaggerated perception may have their genesis in feedback given by other medical specialists.

Finally, there is the declaration-and-challenge, "I have tried everything and nothing helps; exercise make it worse"; "Things will probably get worse"; "My doctor sent me to you to fix my pain" (subtext: "I dare you to try"). Notice how easily exercise is dismissed. Secondary gain issues are likely to playing a large role. These patients frequently present as though they have an unusually close relationship with their other doctors and may even indicate that certain treatments or strong pain medication have been recommended.

Unfortunately, the case of Martha is not an uncommon scenario. The basis of it often lies in unrealistic expectations. It is much easier to manage these at the onset of treatment than after it has commenced. A second, and related, factor is patient responsibility. All too often the patient is inadvertently encouraged to believe that their pain relief is under the control of clinician. They are given medications and procedures are performed on them, without any stipulation of their role and responsibility. Once the situation gets to this point, there is little to do but calmly attempt to redefine the goals and expectations of treatment. Sustained pain relief 24 hours/day and 100% pain relief are goals that cannot be supported by the clinical literature. A 30% to 60% global improvement is generally realistic. It can be useful to engage the patient by asking for their understanding of what they thought to be possible and how they arrived at this. Comparing chronic pain to diabetes can be useful. One can point out the absence of any drug to cure diabetes and that insulin only produces the best results if the patient participate in their own care by exercising, diet, and weight control.

TREATMENT

The 2016 Centers for Disease Control and Prevention (Dowell et al, 2016) report has been high-jacked, as it were, by a number of organizations and agencies and adopted as a rule (see Chapter 22 of this volume). Many clinicians are plagued by repeated contacts all but demanding a reduction the morphine milligram equivalent to at least 90 mg/day if not 50 mg/day or complete tapering of the opioid. The Centers for Disease Control and Prevention report clearly states that it was intended for primary care physicians and that these recommendations did not apply to long-standing (legacy) patients.

Indeed, this report, and subsequent commentaries, have cautioned against "forced" reductions. Nevertheless, many well-controlled, compliant, and functional patients are being compelled to accept lower than effective dosages. In fact, there appears to have been an increase in suicide rate among chronic pain patients placed in this situation. It is not difficult to imagine how devastating and frustrating it would be to the patient and family to be forced to accept a significant reduction in quality of life knowing it could be better and that the change was unrelated to anything they have done. Too often the only defense the clinician can provide is to blame outside agencies. A small, periodic, agreed upon, and temporary reduction as a means of establishing the necessity of the existing dosage is not unreasonable and should be documented in the record.

There is an increasing body of literature supporting the presence of an endogenous opioid system that can influence a broad range of psychological disorders included mood disorders (Sachy, 2010). Unbeknownst to the clinician, the use of opioids in the treatment of chronic pain may help to stabilize an underlying mood disorder, independent of its effect on pain and function. The threat of this returning as a result of reduced dosage can provoke outrage. It is important to carefully monitor and document changes in pain, function, and affect mood, especially in those patients noted to be depressed on the initial consultation.

Some clinicians use the patient's expressed dissatisfaction as an opportunity to "trial" a variety of procedures, knowing full well the likelihood of success in marginal, at best. The possibility of some type of unusual adverse event or side effect, culminating in medical-legal action, should not be underestimated. The approach to this patient should be conservative and involve patient participation (Groves, 1978; Hull et al, 2007). The patient will often self-discharge by failing to keep scheduled appointments when not receiving the medication they want even in the face of acceptable alternative.

Patients with certain personality disorders are driven to create conflict and chaos. They may sabotage their own treatment as a means of engaging the clinician in a debate—one you can never win. It is the demonstration of "control" by engendering such conflict and chaos they find reinforcing. At such times indicating what it is that can, and will, be offered to the patient, and the willingness to refer them to another setting, may be appropriate and the only option (Adams and Murray, 1998).

There will be occasions when such patients are so disruptive to the office that discharge may be necessary. This is frequently met by various accusations of medical malpractice and the threat of a law suit. Box 15.2 outlines steps to take when discharging a patient for the practice. Verbally challenging or attempting to talk over such patients is likely to only escalate the conflict. Sometimes, the best way to win a tug-of-war is to let go of the rope.

At times, the patient's actions may reflect upheaval in other areas of their life (eg, divorce, job lose or dissatisfaction, financial issues, etc.). There is not always the time needed in a busy practice to sort this out. However, just sitting back and allowing the patient to give their narrative for 15 to 20 minutes can be effective. It often provides the basis for some clarification and offering assistance via a referral to a pain psychologist.

BOX 15.2   **Steps to Take When Discharging a Patient**

- Document the interaction thoroughly in the medical record.
- Provide a discharge letter.
- Provide instruction for tapering of medications.
- Offer to transfer records with the appropriate request.
- Indicate where to seek alternative treatment (eg, contacting the local medical society for other pain physician).
- Provide instructions as to seeking emergency care if needed.

- Unrealistic expectations is a common factor among angry and dissatisfied patients. Make sure these are clarified verbally and in writing (eg, the medical agreement) can reduce future problems.
- Some patients—and the reasons vary—are chronically unhappy and dissatisfied. They look for an opportunity to engage in conflict. Debating and arguing is not likely to bring about a solution.
- The clinician must maintain a profession demeanor but be prepared to take decisive action if called for. Efforts should be made to create a mental health referral network.
- There is no substitute for a comprehensive assessment that seeks to identify potentially problematic patients. Instructions as to goals of treatment as well the patient expectation and responsibilities should be part of this process.
- Pain relief is not the only, or perhaps, primary metric of patient satisfaction. The interpersonal aspects of the patient–clinician relationship are critical.

Further Reading

Adams J, Murray R. The general approach to the difficult patient. *Emerg Med Clin North Am.* 1998;16:689–700.

Brown R. Broadening the search for safe treatments in dementia agitation a possible role for low-dose opioids? *Int J Geriatr Psychiatry.* 2010;25:1085–1086.

Bruehl S, Burns JW, Chung OY, Chont M. Pain-related effects of trait anger expression: Neural substrates and the role of endogenous opioid mechanisms. *Neurosci Biobehav Rev.* 2009;33(3):475–491.

Carlson J, Youngblood R, Dalton JA, Blau W, Lindley C. Is patient satisfaction a legitimate outcome of pain management? *J Pain Symptom Manage.* 2003;25(3):264–275.

Comley AL, DeMeyer EJ. Assessing patient satisfaction with pain management through a continuous quality improvement effort. *Pain Symptom Manage.* 2001;21(1):27–40.

Dowell D, Haegerich TM, Chou R. CDC guideline for prescribing opioids for chronic pain—United States. *MMWR Recomm Rep.* 2016;65(1):1–49.

Fan Y, Duncan NW, de Greck M, Northoff G. Is there a core neural network in empathy? An fMRI based quantitative meta-analysis. *Neurosci Biobehav Rev.* 2011;35(3):903–911.

Fernandez E, Wasan A. The anger of pain sufferers: attributions to agents and appraisals of wrongdoing. In: Potegal M, Stemmler G, Spielberger C, eds., *International Handbook of Anger: Constituent and Concomitant Biological, Psychological, and Social Processes.* New York, NY: Springer; 2009:449–464.

Fishbain DA, Bruns D, Disorbio JM, Lewis JE. What are the variables that are associated with the patient's wish to sue his physician in patients with acute and chronic pain? *Pain Med.* 2008;9:1130–1142.

Groves JE. Taking care of the hateful patient. *N Engl J Med.* 1978;296:883–887.

Hirsh AT, Atchison JW, Berger JJ, et al. Patient satisfaction with treatment for chronic pain: Predictors and relationship to compliance. *Clin J Pain.* 2005;21(4):302–310.

Hojat M, Vergare M, Maxwell K, et al. The devil is in the third year: a longitudinal study of erosion of empathy in medical school. *Academic Med.* 2009;84(9):1182–1191.

Husebo BS, Ballard C, Cohen-Mansfield J, Seifert R, Aarsland D. The response of agitated behavior to pain management in persons with dementia. *Am J Geriatr Psychiatry.* 2014;22:708–717.

Hull SH, Broquet K. How to manage difficult patient encounters. *Fam Pract Manag.* 2007;14(6):30–34.

Love TM, Stohler CS, Zubieta JK. Positron emission tomography measures of endogenous opioid neurotransmission and impulsiveness traits in humans. *Arch Gen Psychiatry.* 2009;66:1124–1134.

Manhapra A, Arias AA, Ballantyne JC. The conundrum of opioid tapering in long-term opioid therapy for chronic pain: a commentary. *Subst Abus.* 2018;39(2):152–161. https://doi.org/10.1080/08897077.2017.1381663

Miyamoto Y, Boylan JM, Coe CL, et al. Negative emotions predict elevated Interleukin-6 in the United States but not in Japan. *Brain Behav Immun.* 2013;34:79–85. https://doi.org/10.1016/j.bbi.2013.07.173

Newton, BW. Walking a fine line: is it possible to remain an empathic physician and have a hardened heart? *Front Hum Neurosci.* 2013;7:233:1–12.

Neumann M, Edelhäuser F, Tauschel D, et al. Empathy decline and its reasons: a systematic review of studies with medical students and residents. *Acad Med.* 2011;86(8):996–1009.

Okifuji A, Turk DC, Curran SL. Anger in chronic pain: investigations of anger targets and intensity. *J Psychosom Res.* 1999;47(1):1–12.

Parkoohi PI, Amirzadeh K, Mohabbati V, Abdollahifard G. Satisfaction with chronic pain treatment. *Anesth Pain Med.* 2015;5(4):e23528.

Sachy TH. Use of opioids in pain patients with psychiatric disorders. *Pract Pain Manage.* 2010;10(7):17–26.

Spielberger C. *State-trait anger expression inventory*. Odessa, FL: Psychological Assessment Resources; 1988.

Sullivan MJ, Adams H, Horan S, Maher D, Boland D, Gross R. The role of perceived injustice in the experience of chronic pain and disability: scale development and validation. *J Occup Rehabil*. 2008;18:249–261.

Trost Z, Vangronsveld K, Linton S, Quartana J, Phillip J, Sullivan ML. Cognitive dimensions of anger in chronic pain. *Pain*. 2012;153:515–517.

Zhou Q, Wang H, Schwartz DM, Stoffels M, Park YH, Zhang Y, Yang D, Demirkaya E, Takeuchi M, Tsai WL, Lyons JJ, Yu X, and 29 others. Loss-of-function mutations in TNFAIP3 leading to A20 haploinsufficiency cause an early-onset autoinflammatory disease. *Nature Genet*. 2016;48:67–73.

16 No Way That's My Drug Screen

Myra is a 34-year-old female who is being treated for chronic pelvic pain. She has undergone several surgeries resulting in pain that has both neuropathic and nociceptive components. She is on a moderate dose of opioid with demonstrated improvement in pain and quality of life. During the intake over a year ago, she admitted to "experimenting" with marijuana in her freshman year of college but has not used since. A recent urine drug screen (UDS) was positive for THC. Myra vehemently argues with the results, insisting that "There is no way that is my drug screen." She offers to submit to another screen. She makes threats regarding an attorney if any action is taken on the basis of that screen or if it becomes part of her medical chart.

What do you do now?

BACKGROUND

Performing UDS is about confirming compliance. Compliance, in general, is an issue. A 2003 World Health Organization report (Sabate, 2003) estimated that only 50% of patients take medications as prescribed. A 2006 National Community Pharmacists Association survey (http://www.ncpa.co/adherence/AdherenceReportCard_Full.pdf. Accessed November, 2020) found that 49% forgot to take prescribed medicine, 31% had not filled at least one script, 29% discontinued before the medicine ran out, and 24% took less than the recommended dose. Self-reported adherence, even among healthcare professionals, is poor at 79%. Between 12% and 20% of patients take other people's medicine (Cramer et al, 2008). Studies indicate noncompliance ranging from 9% to 45%: 56% noncompliance for long-term medication versus 22% for short-term medications (see Kidding et al, 2014). In a study of Veterans Administration patients in the primary care setting, the UDS was positive for an illicit drug/unreported opioid in 19.5% of the patients and negative for the prescribed drug in 25.2% (Sekhon et al, 2013).

There are several ways of obtaining information on drug use: urine, blood, hair, and saliva. The UDS is probably the most common approach in general clinical practices. There are two levels of analysis: point-of-care (POC) and confirmatory testing. The most common confirmatory test is the gas chromatography mass spectrometry (GCMS), considered by many to be the gold standard. The POC test is not as sensitive or specific as the GCMS. It should be considered a screen and perhaps the basis for a discussion. However, clinical decisions should be withheld pending the GCMS results.

The more attention you pay to the collection and processing of the UDS, the more likely you will avoid bothersome, if not meaningless, questions or, worse, accusation of an invalid sample/result from the patient. For example, the collection area should be as secure as possible to avoid any question about the authenticity of the specimen. Ideally, the patient should be observed, though this is not practical in most circumstances. Provisions should be made to minimize diluting or contamination of the specimen. Colored water in the commode and the lack of running water (eg, sink) are advised (see Box 16.1).

Chain of custody (CoC) defines a process that must be followed for evidence to be legally defensible. The main elements include that the evidence collector (i) properly identifies the evidence and (ii) is a neutral party who has no personal interest in the test results. A CoC form travels with the specimen, documenting the collection, transfer, receipt, analysis, storage, and disposal of physical and electronic evidence of a drug test. The CoC safeguards the rights of the donor by demonstrating the specimen remained under the control and supervision of the authorized testing personnel. CoC is used mostly in occupational and forensic settings. In most clinic settings, a strict CoC may not be followed, but the security of the specimen must be tightly controlled.

ASSESSMENT

Interpretation of the GCMS testing is important. The lab can give the facts, but the clinician must put the results in context. For example, the absence of a prn opioid is different than if it were prescribed to be take several times a day. Codeine/hydrocodone can be found is some cough medicines (see Table 16.1). A test that is positive for methamphetamine may not represent use of an illicit drug. A d/l isomer assessment is needed. If the specimen contains 20% or more of the d (drug) isomer, the donor is considered positive for an illicit drug. Products such as Vicks inhaler will be associated with the l (legal) isomer. Likewise, testing to confirm the use of alcohol should reveal both ethyl glucuronide (EtG) and ethyl sulfate metabolites. EtG is often seen in patients with diabetes. If the patient's diabetes is uncontrolled, excess glucose in the blood is excreted into the urine and can be fermented into alcohol by microbial organisms.

A Centers for Disease Control and Prevention (2016) report states:

> Clinicians should not test for substances for which results would not affect patient management or for which implications for patient management are unclear. For example, experts noted that there might be uncertainty about the clinical implications of a positive urine drug test for tetrahydrocannabinol (THC).

As of this writing (February 8, 2019), THC is designated as a schedule 1 drug (Cl; Controlled Substance Act, 1970) by the Drug Enforcement Administration (DEA) along with heroine and LSD. C1 drugs are (i) not approved for use in the United States, (ii) considered to have a high abuse potential, and (iii) require a special DEA license to obtain and use for research purposes. Assuming a confirmatory test was carried out revealing the proper metabolite, 11-nor-delta-9-tetrahydrocannabinol-9-carboxylic acid, and potential sources of a false positive are ruled out, the implication is clear: the patient has used an illicit drug as defined by the DEA.

There are many issues regarding this designation, and a majority of states have approved some form of THC or at least decriminalized it. To say it has been "legalized" is a misnomer: state laws can be more but not less restrictive than federal laws. The issue is not with the interpretation of the GCMS drug screen but how the individual clinician chooses to address it. The "don't ask–don't tell" policy may be ill-advised. Individual state medical boards may vary in their approach. The clinician should stay well informed on this matter.

TABLE 16.1. **Drugs and Food That Can Give False Positive Results on Drug Tests**

Drug of Abuse	Cross-Reactive Drug or Food
	Stimulants
Amphetamines	Amantadine
	Phentermine
Cocaine	Coca Leaf Tea
Methamphetamine	Trazodone
	Bupropion
	Desipramine
	Ranitidine
	Selegiline
	Phenylpropanolamine
	Vicks Vapor Inhaler
	Amantadine
	Phentermine
	Opioids
Methadone	Quetiapine
	Chlorpromazine
	Doxylamine
	Diphenhydramine
	Dextromethorphan
Heroin or Morphine	Poppy Seeds
	Rifampin
	Quinolone Antibiotics
	Dextromethorphan
	Hallucinogens
Marijuana/THC	Dronabinol
	Pantoprazole
	Efavirenz
	Hemp Seed
	Benzodiazepines
Diazepam (Valium)	Oxaprozin
Alprazolam (Xanax)	Sertraline
	Barbiturates
Phenobarbitol	Phenytoin
Pentobarbitol	Primidone
	Butalbital

Source: https://fox61.com/2015/03/17/what-drugs-and-food-can-interact-with-urine-testing/.

The window of detection can vary. A single use of marijuana is detectable in the urine for 3 to 7 days; moderate use is detectable for 5 to 7 days, daily use for 10 to 15 days, and long-term/heavy use for over a month. The strength of the drug and the body composition of the user play a role as THC is absorbed in fatty tissue. Second-hand smoke is a debatable issue. Most believe it could only occur under extreme environmental circumstances and is detectable only within hours of exposure. If a patient were to argue the case, at the very least they could be could be held accountable for poor decision-making regarding the company they keep and the risk of diversion questioned. If the presence of the substance is confirmed, the patient should be questioned as to how something they claim not to have taken could possibly be in their system. A satisfactory response is not likely, but the patient understands the predicament their denial has caused.

The detection time for alcohol is 3 to 4 days and for cocaine 1 to 4 days. Depending on the regularity and randomness of the UDS, a moderate marijuana user's use of alcohol and cocaine could go undetected. The landscape on this matter is shifting rapidly. Because the prime objective of the clinician is the protection of society by preventing diversion, a conservative approach may warrant consideration.

TREATMENT

The cause(s) for noncompliance or aberrant drug behavior vary. These can include addiction, psychiatric comorbidity (impulsiveness/personality disorder, depression, anxiety, etc.), cognitive dysfunction, and/or criminal intent (diversion). Aberrant behavior does not equal addiction. It is a matter of type and extent (Passik and Kirsh, 2004). One study demonstrated as many as 45% of chronic pain patients produced an abnormal UDS; 20% showed illicit drugs. Young age was the only predictive variable (Michna and Jamison, 2007). A second study (Schnider and Mill, 2012) found an inconsistent UDS 15.4% of the time. Patients with inconsistent UDS were questioned. One individual was positive for amphetamine, which was being prescribed by a psychiatrist. In another case, the POC UDS was positive for amphetamines but negative on GCMS confirmation. It is critical to have an updated and accurate list of all medications taken by a patient.

Noncompliance is not a contemporary problem. Indeed, Balfour and Smellie quote from a 1778 publication stating

> Such patients are to be expelled from the infirmary: (1) Who at their admission falsified their disease; or intentionally concealed any material part of it. (2) Who refuse the food, drink, medicines, or operations prescribed, or take any medicines, drink, or food, not ordered by the physicians or surgeons. (p. 342)

Some clinicians opt to summarily discharge any patient producing a UDS suggestive of noncompliance with the medical agreement. Although understandable, this approach may be a bit draconian. As noted earlier, there may be viable explanations. Others are more inclined to give a warning. Depending upon the circumstances (eg, a patient with a long history of compliance, an excellent response to opioid therapy, and/or a reasonable explanation), this may prevent a patient from having to seek treatment elsewhere. Finding a new clinician would be difficult if it were known that they were discharged for noncompliance. Finally, some clinicians adapt the philosophy of "discharge the molecule, not the patient." That is, offer noncontrolled substances and nondrug therapies. This gives the patient the opportunity to reestablish a sense of trust.

An inconsistent UDS can provide a basis for a teaching moment. Educating the patient on the implication if it were to occur in a legal context, such as after an accident, can help them to understand the seriousness of the matter. It can be used to discuss a potential addiction problem along with treatment alternatives. This could include a requirement to participate in psychological counseling and/or some form of rehabilitation therapy.

The magnitude of the infraction also plays a role. It is one thing to have a UDS positive for alcohol but quite another for heroine. If the patient is discharged, a letter should be given to the patient or sent by certified mail. Ideally, it should give recommendations for therapy and advice to seek medical attention in the event of any complications. Indeed, one should be very cautious about prescribing opioids in the presence of a confirmatory UDS for illicit substances.

KEY POINTS TO REMEMBER

- Interpreting drug screens is deceptively simple yet endlessly complex.
- The clinician would be well-served to have a working relationship with the pharmacologist at the lab performing the confirmatory testing.
- Maintain a current and signed medical agreement that outlines possible consequences for noncompliance. Leave yourself some "wiggle room" by using terms like could, will consider, may, and so on.
- Remember that the only thing worse than not having a medical agreement is not following the one you have.
- Make decisions within the context of your background, experience, and available support.
- Those in a one-person practice may have to be more conservative than those in a multidisciplinary setting.
- Attention to procedure details up front can save future time and energy.
- Your decision should involve deliberation and consideration of the context and consequences. When in doubt, go with the science.

Further Reading

Dowell D, Haegerich TM, Chou R. CDC guideline for prescribing opioids for chronic pain—United States. MMWR Recomm Rep. 2016;65(1):1–49.

Cramer JA, Benedict A, Muszbek N, Keskinaslan A, Khan M. The significance of compliance and persistence in the treatment of diabetes, hypertension and dyslipidaemia: a review. Int J Clin Pract. 2008;62(1):76–87.

Kipping K, Maier C, Bussemas HH, Schwarzer A. Medication compliance in patients with chronic pain. Pain Physician. 2014;17:81–94.

Michna E, Jamison R, Pham L, Ross E, Janfaza D, Nedeljkovic S, Narang S, Palombi D, Wasan A. Urine toxicology among chronic pain patients on opioid therapy: frequency and predictability of abnormal findings. Clin J Pain. 2007;23:173–179.

Passik SD, Kirsh KL. Opioid therapy in patients with a history of substance abuse. CNS Drugs. 2004;18:13–25.

Sabate E (ed). *Adherence to long-term therapies: Evidence for action.* Geneva, Switzerland: WHO, 2003.

Schneider JP, Miller A. Urine drug tests in a private chronic pain practice. *Pract Pain Manag.* 2012;8(1): 1–4.

Sekhon R, Aminjavahery N, Davis CN, Roswarski MJ, Robinette C. Compliance with opioid treatment guidelines for chronic non-cancer pain (CNCP) in primary care at a Veterans Affairs Medical Center (VAMC). *Pain Med.* 2013;14(10):1548–1556.

The History and Statutes of the Royal Infirmary of Edinburgh. Edinburgh, England: E. Balfour and Smellie; 1778:76–77. Cited in *BMJ.* 2004;328:342.

17 The Abandoned Patient

Scenario 1: Joe has been treated by Dr. R.M. for several years. His opioid dose has been escalated to include a 100 ug fentanyl patch every 48 hours along with oxycodone 15 mg qid for breakthrough pain. Although he claims some relief, he has increased symptoms prior to the end of the 48 hours. For reasons that are unclear, Dr. R.M. has given notice that he will no longer be prescribing pain medication and that patients need to find an alternative. Joe presents to your office pleading his case and noting he will be out of medicine in 10 days.

Scenario 2: Joe has been treated by a pain management physician for several years, receiving interventional therapy and medications. Upon arriving for his regular appointment, he is greeted with a notice on the door that interventions will still be available but pain medications will no longer be prescribed. Joe is a given a final prescription for one month and will soon be out.

Scenario 3: Joe was recently relocated from a neighboring state by his employer. He has a prescription from his previous pain management physician but is unable to get it filled locally. He will soon run out of medicine and is fearful of going through withdrawal.

What do you do now?

BACKGROUND

Pain management, especially as it relates to the use of opioids for chronic pain, has had an interesting history. A variety of opioid medications, including opium and morphine, were readily available, often as over-the-counter preparations, beginning in the 1800s. The Harrison Narcotics Tax Act of 1914 was implemented to regulate the production and sale of opioids due to concerns relating to addiction. Opioid addiction declined in the 1920s. The Controlled Substance Act of 1970 established a federal U.S. drug policy under which the manufacture, importation, possession, use, and distribution of certain substances is regulated. This legislation created a five-category system based, in part, on the abuse potential of the substance. The Drug Enforcement Administration and Food and Drug Administration (FDA) determined how a drug was to be classified.

Several papers appeared in the 1980s written by palliative care physicians encouraging the long-term use of opioids. A retrospective study by Portenoy and Foley (1986) reported effective management in 38 noncancer pain patients; 73% used about 20 milligrams morphine equivalents (MME) per day and demonstrated a low risk of iatrogenic addiction. This report helped to usher in an age of opioid prescribing for chronic noncancer pain. Agencies and societies such as the Federation of State Medical Boards, the Joint Commission Accreditation of Healthcare Organizations, the American Pain Society (APS), and the American Academy of Pain Medicine supported and created guidelines for the use of opioids. Concerns over the under (inadequate) treatment of cancer-related pain generalized to noncancer pain. In 1995, the APS introduced the Pain as the 5th Vital Sign campaign, promoting increased assessment and treatment of pain. A similar position was adopted by the Veteran's Health Administration in 1988.

It soon became apparent that opioids were being prescribed at levels well above those reported by Portenoy and Foley. This was made easier by the availability of more potent and longer acting opioids. By 2010 increased opioid-related deaths, diversion, and addiction were noted. A 2016 Centers for Disease Control and Prevention (CDC) report (Dowell et al, 2016) outlined existing literature and recommendations, which, although intended for the primary care physician, were adopted by many agencies, state medical boards, and insurance companies as a general policy. Indeed, the American Medical Association, the American College of Surgeons, The Joint Commission, the American Academy of Family Physicians, and the Centers for Medicare and Medicaid services eventually withdrew their advocacy of the Pain as the 5th Vital Sign campaign (Levy et al, 2018) recognizing that opioid prescribing, especially in the hospital setting, based on a subjective verbal report of pain and wherein patient "satisfaction" was judged by patient-reported pain relief contributed to the overuse of opioids.

Many physicians began to feel both perceived and real pressure to reconsider their prescribing criteria and habits. Law enforcement stepped up its pursuit and prosecution of physicians committing fraudulent and illegal acts involving opioids. The backlash was a sudden reduction and discontinuation of opioid use, especially for chronic pain, on the part of many physicians. The situation reached such a level in 2019 that agencies began to issue cautionary notes about overly aggressive opioid tapering (see Kolodny et al, 2015, for greater detail).

The three scenarios presented at the beginning of this chapter have become increasingly common since the release of the CDC report in 2016. In some cases, such as scenario 1, an "aggressive" prescriber became very wary and simply abandoned the patient to their own resources. Some interventionists were limited in the scope of their practice and no longer provided medication management. There have been instances where medications were prescribed only if the patient consented to interventional therapy as well. Some primary care physicians, out of apparent fear of sanctions, are discontinuing the use of opioids, even at small doses (20 MME or less). A significant number of legitimate patients with chronic pain patients are being displaced, through no fault of their own. They often present in a state of desperation secondary to existing or pending dire circumstances (ie, opioid withdrawal).

ASSESSMENT

A 1992 report from the Agency for Health Care Policy and Research asserted the "ethical obligation to manage pain and relieve the patient's suffering is at the core of a health care professional's commitment" (p. 25). This obligation places the ethical clinician in a bind when faced with the patient who has been "abandoned." In general, existing guidelines do not expect the clinician to simply continue what has been started. The patient should be treated as a new patient to the clinical setting.

The patient will present with, and the clinician is likely feel, a sense of urgency. However, shortcuts should be avoided. A proper assessment including examination, drug screen, and Prescription Drug Monitoring Program check need to be done. When possible, one should contact the previous prescriber to confirm the patient's story. Be careful about providing a "bridge prescription." Patients should be informed of their options if they experience withdrawal symptoms prior to you assuming care. These might include hospitals or centers equipped to handle such situations. Patients may play on your sympathies, become insistent or even threatening, or make accusations of you lacking concern. This is especially likely if their former prescriber referred them to you. Remember, once you prescribe, you have forged a doctor-patient relationship. Information documenting patients' treatment history and compliance is critical.

One may, and perhaps should, feel obligated to help manage pain, but you are not obligated to do anything listed in Box 17.1.

A liberal prescriber quickly becomes known among those seeking opioids for legitimate and nonlegitimate reasons. A practice can become the epicenter for undesirable patients. Such patients are more likely to sell, swap, or trade their prescriptions; even in the parking lot. A full parking lot early in the morning, cars from out of state, an office full of sedated patients, and individuals "hanging around" are red flags for the authorities.

BOX 17.1 **You Are Not Obligated To**

- Prescribe on the first visit.
- Treat in the absence of an adequate diagnostic workup (physical/psychological).
- Treat with opioids.
- Treat as the patient specifies.
- Use only pharmacological therapies.
- Treat without requiring patient involvement and responsibility.

TREATMENT

The current climate has produced a heightened interest in tapering opioids (see Chapter 22 of this volume). When confronted with any of the scenarios presented in this chapter, the clinician has at least three choices. First, the clinician can direct the appropriate patient to a medically assisted treatment (MAT) program. Or, if trained and certified, they can initiate MAT. Second, after gathering sufficient baseline information, the clinician can initiate a tapering program. Several such programs have been described (Darnell et al, 2012; Sullivan et al, 2017). The rate of reduction varies from 10% to 25% per month, based on drug and patient tolerance. The CDC provides a very concise "Pocket Guide: Tapering Opioids for Chronic Pain" (www.cdc.gov/drugoverdose/prescribing/guideline.html). Third, the patient can be referred to a facility providing the needed services.

If the clinician feels compelled to help, and has sufficient information to initiate prescribing, it is best to do so only if the patient is taking, or willing to take, a level of opioid the clinician is experienced with and agrees to the medication agreement. These patients should be monitored more carefully and seen more frequently until a pattern of compliance and effectiveness is established or confirmed. Some clinicians feel this is an opportunity, and are more comfortable, shifting the patient to a buprenorphine product, such as Belbuca® or Burtrans Patch®. Both appear to be effective and as Schedule III drugs are considered safer with less potential for abuse. As they are FDA approved for pain, they do not carry the same implications or stigma as Suboxone®, which is approved for substance use disorder.

Although not necessarily "abandoning" patient, many surgeons have limited the amount and type of postsurgical medications they will prescribe. Evidence suggests that up to 13% of opioid-naive patients continue to take opioids long after postsurgical care is completed (Clarke et al, 2014).

Indeed, one healthcare organization has identified this prolonged narcotic usage as a "hospital-acquired condition and should be considered a question of patient safety" (HealthTrust, 2017). A number of preoperative, intraoperative, and postoperative risk factors have been identified (Chapman and Vierchy, 2017; Clarke et al, 2014). Tapering and reassessing the postoperative patient is a recommended strategy (Clarke et al, 2018).

Patients will exhibit a good deal of fear and trepidation at the thought of tapering off their opioid medication. At times this is the medically prudent approach. Even if done at a patient's request, the outcome is variable. A recent article (Goesling et al, 2019) reported half of the patients requesting cessation of opioids secondary to lack of effect, fear of addition, and impact of quality of life rated their pain as unchanged or better. The other half reported increased pain following opioid cessation. The authors stated that "As the pendulum swings from pain control to drug control, we must ensure that the response to the opioid epidemic does not cause harm to individuals with chronic pain" (p. 1131). A similar report involving patients treated for chronic noncancer pain at the Veterans Administration found that over 53% of patients reported their pain to be "moderate or severe" following removal of their opioid therapy (McPerson et al, 2018). There may be a subgroup of patients who are compliant, cooperative, and opioid-responsive. One must be alert to this possibility and protective of these patients (Kertesz, 2016, 2017).

KEYS POINTS TO REMEMBER

- Sooner or later, every clinician will encounter the patient who has been abandoned.
- Be cautious about short-cutting your usual intake process.
- Have a list of referral sources on hand.
- Be careful of the patient with the fewest records, sketchiest history, and loudest demands.

Further Reading

Agency for Health Care Policy and Research. The US Department of Health and Human Services. Publication # 92-0032. *Clinical guidelines on acute pain management*. Rockville, MD; Feb. 1992.

Chapman CR, Vierchy CJ. The transition of acute postoperative pain to chronic pain: an integrative overview of research on mechanisms. *J Pain*. 2017;18(4):359. e1-359.e38.

Clarke H, Azargive S, Montbriand J, et al. Opioid weaning and pain management in postsurgical patients at the Toronto General Hospital Transitional Pain Service. *Can J Pain*. 2018;2(1):236–247.

Clarke H, Soneji N, Ko DT, Yun L, Wijeysundera DN. Rates and risk factors for prolonged opioid use after major surgery: population based cohort study. *BMJ*. 2014;348:g1251.

Darnall BD, Stacey BR, Chou R. Medical and psychological risks and consequences of long-term opioid therapy in women. *Pain Med*. 2012;13(9):1181–1211.

Dowell D, Haegerich TM, Chou R. CDC guideline for prescribing opioids for chronic pain—United States. *MMWR Recomm Rep*. 2016;65(1):1–49.

Goesling J, DeJonckheere M, Pierce J, Williams DA, Brummett C, Hassett A, Clauw DJ. Opioid cessation and chronic pain: perspectives of former opioid users. *Pain*. 2019;160(5):1131–1145.

HealthTrust. Perioperative Pain Management Collaboration Summit. Nashville, TN; 2017, Apr. 12–13.

Kertesz SG. *Opioids, addiction and pain: message clarity to prevent harm and save lives. briefing for policy leaders*. 2017. https://media.lasvegasnow. com/nxsglobal/lasvegasnow/document_dev/2017/10/19/Briefing%20for%20 Leaders%20%20%202-18-2017update_1508448667952_28033936_ver1.0.pdf. Accessed November, 2020.

Kertesz SG. Turning the tide or riptide? The changing opioid epidemic. *Subst Abuse*. 2017;38(1):3–8. doi:10.1080/08897077.2016.1261070

Kolodny A, Courtwright DT, Hwang CS, Kreiner P, Eadie JL, Clark TW, Alexander GC. The prescription opioid and heroin crisis: a public health approach to an epidemic of addiction. *Ann Rev Public Health*. 2015;36:559–574.

Levy N, Sturgess J, Mills P. "Pain as the fifth vital sign" and dependence on the "numerical pain scale" is being abandoned in the US: why? *Br J Anaesth*. 2018;120(3):435–438.

McPherson S, Smith CL, Dobscha S, Morasco B, Demidenko MI, Meath THA, Lovejoy T. Changes in pain intensity after discontinuation of long-term opioid therapy for chronic noncancer pain. *Pain*. 2018;159(10):2097–2104.

Sullivan MD, Turner JA, DiLodovico C, D'Appollonio A, Stephens K, Chan YF. Prescription opioid taper support for outpatients with chronic pain: a randomized controlled trial. *J Pain*. 2017;18(3):308–318.

18 The Not-So-Perfect Remedy

JD is a 52-year-old male complaining of pain in his right foot/ankle following a work-related injury. He had an open reduction internal fixation with subsequent removal of displaced hardware. He is a longtime user of cigarettes and used cannabis is delta-9 (Δ9) delta tetrahydrocannabinol (THC) daily in the past. He claims to have nightmares and flashbacks. He never returned to work and was awarded social security disability. He has been on long-term medication management but in the last year began having urine drug screens (UDSs) positive for THC. He claims it must be secondary to the cannabidiol (CBD) product he is using. He also reports the CBD helps his pain, reduced the need for pain medications and improvement in sleep, anxiety, and posttraumatic stress disorder symptoms. Although he reportedly has discontinued the product, THC is found in subsequent UDSs.

"Doc, I am not sure what all the fuss is about. Okay, so there is THC in my drug screen. After all, it is legal in the majorities of states, and it does help many of my symptoms including pain. I understand that you may not want to prescribe it, but I do not see why it should affect other medications you are giving me."

What do you do now?

BACKGROUND

The Controlled Substances Act (CSA) of 1970 made marijuana a Schedule I drug, along with LSD and heroin, and declared it had no medicinal value and a high potential for abuse; this designation has not changed as of 2020. It is, however, important to have some understanding about the complexity of the cannabis plant and its constituent parts.

Marijuana (aka cannabis, weed, herb, pot, grass, bud, ganja) refers to the dried leaves, flowers, stems, and seeds from the Cannabis Sativa or Cannabis Indica plant. The primary psychoactive component of cannabis is THC. The terms *THC* and *marijuana* are often used interchangeably. But, in fact, THC is only one of the 483 known compounds in the plant.

The plant contains a large number of cannabinoids. Cannabinoids are various naturally occurring, biologically active, chemical constituents (eg, CBD and cannabinol) of cannabis. There are at least 113 different cannabinoids isolated from cannabis, exhibiting varying effects. Cannabis oil (butane honey oil, shatter, wax, and crumble), which can be smoked or vaporized by pressing the extracted oil against the heated surface of an oil rig pipe (dabbing), may contain up to 75% Δ9 THC versus 5% to 20% in the herb or resin.

Endocannabinoid system. The reason any of these compounds have any effect at all is based on the existence of the endocannabinoid system (ECS), in the same way that opioid pain medicines have their effect because of the presence of an endogenous opioid system. The ECS went undiscovered until the 1990s. The uncovering of the chemical structures, and the synthesizing of cannabinoids, were the catalysts for further research on both animals and humans that led to the discovery of cannabinoid receptors in the 1980s and an ECS in the 1990s (Pertwee, 2006).

ECS is a biological system within the human body that is composed of endocannabinoids. The ECS system is a key homeostatic regulator in the body. The ECS consists of a series of receptors configured to react to endocannabinoids, phytocannabinoids (eg, THC and other compounds found in a variety of plants, including cannabis), and synthetic cannabinoids. The two primary endocannabinoids are anandamide (AEA) and 2-arachidonoylglycerol (2-AG). AEA and 2-AG have binding affinity to two G-protein receptors, CB1 and CB2.

This system is involved in energy intake, nutrient transport, and metabolism storage. It is also thought to be involved in regulating a variety of physiological and cognitive processes, including various activity of the immune system, pain sensation, mood, and memory (Aizpurua-Olaizola et al, 2017; Pandey et al, 2009; Donvito et al, 2017). Therefore, ECS subserves a whole host of functions, beyond that involving THC and other related cannabis products. Indeed, ECS is often considered to be of importance comparable to that of the nervous system in general.

Injury, disease, and illness can promote the release of proinflammatory cytokines. Once the need for proinflammatory cytokines has ceased, the ECS negative feedback loop can override cellular signaling from lymphatic, endocrine, or other systems involved in the healing process. This may help prevent the ongoing release of proinflammatory substances known to play a role in chronic, especially neuropathic, pain and hyperalgesia.

Delta-9 delta tetrahydrocannabinol. THC is perhaps the most potent and most studied of the cannabinoids (Hazekamp Grotenhermen, 2010). It was isolated in the 1960s. Specific cannabinoid receptors CB1 and CB2 were discovered in the early 1990s. CB1 receptors are located primarily in the brain in areas associated with higher mental functions, memory/cognition, and movement, as well as areas associated with anxiety, pain, sensory perception, motor coordination, and endocrine function. CB1 receptors tend to inhibit the release of neurotransmitters such as acetylcholine, glutamate, norepinephrine, dopamine, serotonin, and gamma–aminobutyric acid (GABA). CB2 receptors are located primarily in the periphery. They influence activity in the immune system and peripheral nerves. CB2 receptors also play an instrumental role in inflammatory reactions. THC triggers dopaminergic neurons in the ventral tegmental area of the brain, a region known to mediate reinforcing (rewarding) effects. This dopaminergic drive is thought to underlie the reinforcing and addicting properties of this drug.

Cannabidiol. CBD is a major constituent of the cannabis plant and the most abundant cannabinoid in hemp. The differences in CBD oil and hemp oil are given in Table 18.1. It does not appear to act directly on CB1 or CB2 receptors. Rather, CBD is a known agonist of serotonin 5-HT1A receptors (Russo et al, 2005) and transient receptor potential vanilloid type 1 receptors (Bisogno et al, 2001). It is also known to enhance adenosine receptor signaling by inhibiting adenosine inactivation. This property may

TABLE 18.1. Comparison of CBD Oil Versus Hemp Oil

Hemp Extract	Hemp Seed Extract
Extracted from whole hemp plant (including leaves, stalk, bud, and flowers)	Extracted from the hemp seed only
Low THC (<0.3%)	No THC
Rich in CBD	No CBD
Can contain additional cannabinoids	Rich in omega 3 and omega 6
Primarily used for medical purposes	Used in cooking, as a topical moisturizer, and as a daily health supplement

THC, tetrahydrocannabinol; CBD, cannabidiol.

be responsible for its potential benefit in treating pain and inflammation (Carrier et al, 2006).

Hemp. Hemp is different from marijuana in its function, cultivation, and application (Table 18.2). Nevertheless, hemp was grouped with all forms of cannabis as a Schedule I drug, as defined in 1970 under the CSA. However, the Hemp Farming Act of 2018 legalized industrial hemp, which

TABLE 18.2. Comparison of Hemp Versus Marijuana

Type	Cannabis	Chemical Makeup	Psychoactive	Cultivation	Applications
Hemp	Yes	Low THC (<0.3%)	No	Can grow with minimal care. Climate friendly	Automobiles, body care, clothing, construction, food, plastic, etc.
Marijuana	Yes	High THC (5%–30% +)	Yes	Grows in carefully controlled atmosphere	Medical and recreational use

THC, tetrahydrocannabinol.

has a THC concentration of no more than 0.3%, effectively removing industrial hemp from the Schedule I classification.

Hemp is a strain of the cannabis plant grown specifically for industrial use (eg, industrial hemp). Indeed, industrial hemp has been shown to have hundreds of potential applications. Although closely related to cannabis, it is a very different crop and is grown in a different way. Industrial hemp farmers grow the plants taller versus regular cannabis plants, as the value of industrial hemp is primarily in its stalk rather than the leaves. Hemp can be used in variety of ways that marijuana cannot. These include dietary supplements, skin products, clothing, and accessories. Hemp products are available online, in grocery stores, and at retail stores.

Terpenes. Terpenes are aroma molecules produced by all plants and are common constituents of flavorings and fragrances found in essential oils (Booth et al, 2017). The cannabis plant contains about 140 of these. Terpenes are made in the trichomes of the plant. Trichomes are the shiny, sticky, mushroom-shaped crystals that cover the leaves and buds and that act as a defense mechanism, protecting the plant from insects and animals by producing fragrant terpenes that repel these dangers (González-Burgos and Gómez-Serranillos, 2012).

Terpenes act on receptors and neurotransmitters. They tend to combine with, or dissolve in, lipids (fats). They function as serotonin uptake inhibitors and can increase norepinephrine and dopamine activity, much like many antidepressants. Terpenes can also augment GABA. Some of the more common terpenes include myrcene, which has anti-inflammatory, analgesic, and sedative properties; pinene, which is energy-enhancing and used as an antibacterial/antimicrobial and for parasite control; and limonene, which can serve to enhance mood, treat antireflux disease, and neutralize stomach acids. Terpenes have been recognized as safe by the Food and Drug Administration (FDA).

Flavonoids. Flavonoids are one of the largest nutrient families known, containing over 6,000 compounds. About 20 of these compounds have been identified in the cannabis plant. Flavonoids are known to have antioxidant and anti-inflammatory properties. Some flavonoids extracted from the cannabis plant have been found to possess pharmacological effects. The role of flavonoids is unclear. They may interact synergistically with cannabinoids to enhance their effects or reduce them (Panche et al, 2017).

ASSESSMENT

It is important to separate out the CBD from the THC user. The labeling of these products is notoriously inaccurate. Bonn-Miller et al (2017) examined CBD products sold as "THC free." With respect to CBD content, 43% of the products were underlabeled, 26% were overlabeled, and 31% were accurate. Regarding vaporization liquids, 87% were mislabeled. Concentration of unlabeled cannabinoids was generally low, and THC was detected in 21% of samples. A UDS with confirmatory testing (see Chapter 16) is needed. The cut-off detection level is important, especially in states where THC is considered illegal. If too low, THC will be detected in a patient using a CBD/hemp product containing the acceptable level (<0.3% THC).

A 2016 Centers for Disease Control and Prevention report stated

> Clinicians should not test for substances for which results would not affect patient management or for which implications for patient management are unclear . . . experts noted that there might be uncertainty about the clinical implications of a positive urine drug test for tetrahydrocannabinol (THC). (p. 31)

Therefore, a fundamental question is the consequence of a positive THC UDS. For some prescribers, THC is an illicit drug that, if present in a UDS, could result in discontinuing or substantially altering treatment. For others, it is of little consequence other than perhaps to confirm compliance.

The laws governing the use of medical marijuana' vary dramatically in their scope (https://public.findlaw.com/cannabis-law/cannabis-laws-and-regulations/medical-marijuana-laws-by-state.html). Some states only allow terminally ill patients to legally use marijuana, while others have an exhaustive list of qualifying illnesses. Patients using physician-prescribed medical marijuana for appropriate illnesses/chronic conditions are exempt from criminal prosecution in states that have passed medical marijuana laws. However, the prescribing clinician, as is the case with any prescribed drug, may have legal exposure. Therefore, in situations where it matters, it may important to identify the patient with an addiction/substance use disorder (SUD; see Chapter 7).

The use of hemp/CBD is another matter. Here it is important to determine the contents of the product. While a confirmatory UDS, especially with a cut-off detection level, may identify those products containing THC, it will not reveal what other component may be present (Bonn-Miller et al, 2017). This can be approximated by obtaining the results of independent laboratory testing. If not available upon request, the patient may be best advised to not use that particular product.

Manufacturers have made various claims of effectiveness. In many cases, the claims are exaggerated and unsupported by any scientific research. The patient and clinician should identify the problem(s) they hope to treat as objectively as possible. The effect of many of these products is fairly immediate. Use of questionnaires, report from reliable significant others, and reduction of other prescribed medication can be used to document effectiveness.

The clinician needs to be aware, and monitor, the patient for THC-related consequences including acute toxicity resulting in difficulty with coordination, decreased muscle strength, decreased hand steadiness, postural hypotension, lethargy, decreased concentration, slowed reaction time, slurred speech, and conjunctival injection. Large doses of THC may produce confusion, amnesia, delusions, hallucinations, anxiety, and agitation, even though most of these episodes remit rapidly. Long-term users may experience paranoia, panic disorder, fear, or dysphoria. A 2020 cross-sectional analyses involving nearly 1,700 THC users (Sturgeon et al, 2020) reported poorer sleep and pain intensity/emotional distress/physical and social dysfunction in patients presenting for the treatment of chronic pain compared to nonusers. A 2020 cross-sectional study reported that the children of mothers using cannabis during pregnancy have a higher incidence of psychopathology in middle childhood (Paul et al, 2020).

Although generally considered to be safe, CBD has been associated with a number of side effects including drowsiness and fatigue, restlessness, headaches, changes in appetite, dry mouth, nausea, lower blood pressure, increased tremors in Parkinson's disease, and euphoria. These are usually mild and reversible. One needs to be cautious about using CBD in combination with nonsteroidal anti-inflammatory drugs, antidepressants, antiepileptic drugs, and anticoagulants (Iffland and Grotenhermen, 2017).

TREATMENT

The National Academies of Science, Engineering, and Medicine issued a report titled *The Health Effects of Cannabis and Cannabinoids,* which was published in book form in 2017. It is a very objective approach to the analysis of the literature up to that time. The report provides the summary shown in Box 18.1.

Delta-9 delta tetrahydrocannabinol. The approach to treatment using THC is likely to be geographically dependent. Some states have fairly liberal laws and have legalized recreational and medical marijuana. For example, marijuana was legalized for medicinal and recreational use by Colorado in 2012. This event attracted significant attention and was called the "great experiment." Pundits on both sides of the issue have carefully observed the outcome. According to a 2018 statement by Kevin Sabet, president of the bipartisan group Smart Approaches to Marijuana, "The state is *not* better off with legal pot" (Measuring Colorado's 'great experiment,'" 2017). It is interesting that, in Colorado, the number of registered medical marijuana users decreased by about 23% from 2014 to 2018. Presumably, registrants abandoned the program to avoid the regulatory hurdles, including visiting their physician every year and the $25 application-processing fee. Buying it at retail stores was more convenient.

Much is yet to be learned about appropriate candidates, appropriate target symptoms, the most effective dosage/delivery system, and how long it should be used. Furthermore, in the setting of chronic pain, what guidelines will be employed regarding the co-utilization with benzodiazepines and alcohol? Even though alcohol is legal throughout the country, most, if not all, guidelines recommend against the use of alcohol with opioids. Will one accept THC as an "opioid-sparing" substance or prohibit co-utilization?

What constitutes a "standard" dose of THC remains unclear. The typical joint size in the United States is 0.66 g, and the average potency is 8% THC, resulting in an average dose of 8.25 mg THC per joint. Occasional users report feeling "high" after consuming only 2 to 3 mg of THC. THC levels ranging from 15% to 20% or higher would yield a THC dose between 9.9 and 13.2 mg. Washington State and Colorado have set the standard dose of THC at 10 mg, while Oregon set its limit at 5 mg. When considering any agent for medical or therapeutic use, one has to answer three questions: Who is the right person, what is the right dose, and for how long should it be used? These questions remain unanswered, even in the states that have legalized recreational and medical marijuana.

Chronic users of THC may experience paranoia, panic disorder, fear, or dysphoria. Transient psychotic episodes may also occur with cannabis use. These psychiatric effects may be less likely to occur with strains that contain higher concentrations of CBD. Ventricular tachycardia has been association THC. A recent review of the literature (Ghasemiesfe et al, 2019) found an increased risk of testicular germ cell tumor among regular users of THC.

Nearly 7% to 10% of regular users become behaviorally and physically dependent on cannabis. Furthermore, early onset of use and daily/weekly use correlates with future dependence. According to the National Institute on Drug Abuse, 100,000 people are treated annually for primary (may be self-perceived) marijuana abuse. In humans, the withdrawal syndrome is not well characterized. Withdrawal symptoms may occur after as little as one week of use.

CBD/hemp: full-spectrum hemp extracts. There are more than 100 active cannabinoids in the cannabis plant. Various preparations (strains) produce various effects. Some have suggested that a pharmacological synergy may exist among these compounds, resulting in an "entourage effect." Therefore, the inclusion of many of the plant's constituents may allow for a greater therapeutic benefit at significantly lower concentrations. The theory of an entourage effect is largely unsubstantiated by research (Booth and Bohlman, 2019).

Broad-spectrum hemp extracts. Broad-spectrum extracts are intermediate, between full-spectrum and isolated products. In the manufacturing of broad-spectrum extracts, only THC is removed. As such, the end user may take advantage of the perceived entourage effect without fear of violating any legal, medical, or job-related regulations.

Isolated cannabinoids. CBD has been shown to be a powerful antiemetic, anti-inflammatory, and antianxiety agent, without exerting a psychotropic effect. CBD has been shown to activate the central nervous system's limbic and paralimbic regions, reducing autonomic arousal and feelings of anxiety. Potential benefits in the treatment of neuropathic pain, hypertension, poststroke neuroprotection, multiple sclerosis, epilepsy, and cancer are being investigated. The benefits of isolated cannabinoids as dietary supplements include (i) higher concentrations of cannabinoids with potential benefits and (ii) exclusion of THC for end users who may be routinely screened or practitioners who have concerns about THC recommendations. The average daily dose of CBD can range from 1 to 6 mg/10 lbs of body weight. However, one study reported doses of up to 1500/day were well tolerated (Greydanus et al, 2013).

Cannabidiol. CBD is being sold in many forms, including pills, tinctures (liquids taken as purchased or mixed with a beverage), isolate (fine crystals, which can be mixed with oils, lotions, food, beverages), topical, vaping

TABLE 18.3. **Clinical Survey Results**

Benefit	Count
Reduced pain/inflammation	16
Reduced anxiety	11
Relaxation	6
Sleep quality	7
Sleep onset	3

pens, and gummies. Delivery systems also vary. XStraw™ is a relatively new oral delivery system with special application for the elderly and pediatric population. The granulated substance (eg, CBD or THC) is premeasured and positioned in a straw-like container. The user removes a straw from the sealed single pack, places it into a drink, and ingests the contents. Pricing of these CBD products also varies widely. The best way to compare is to determine the cost per milligram of CBD.

An informal survey of a group of 44 patients in our clinic who have been using a product containing a standardized dose of 25 mg of CBD from hemp oil extract for 6 months or more are shown in Table 18.3. Reduction in pain and anxiety were most commonly reported. None of the patients reported any adverse reactions.

Of the individuals who reported benefit, over 50% had some diagnosis of musculoskeletal pain, with low back pain being the most prevalent followed by neck pain. Nerve-related pain represented a significantly smaller percentage of diagnoses but was still present in several respondents. The results of this survey are inconclusive but are supportive of the literature review presented in Box 18.1.

CLINICAL CASES

There are at least three responses to the cases in this chapter. The first is, "Sorry, I will not give any controlled substance if you are positive for THC." The second is, "Okay, but I am going to reduce the dosage of your opioids."

The third is, "I never expected that THC would resolve your pain. We will continue with our treatment plan as long as you continue to be functional and adhere to the agreement."

In the case of JD, one must be suspicious of an SUD. He is being treated in a state where no provisions have been made for the use of medical marijuana. He is aware that use of THC is prohibited by the medical agreement. Although having been counseled about the issue, he has committed further violations. He has a history of THC use. Continued use of opioids may well be questioned by the medical board, and knowingly prescribing these may increase the clinician's liability and legal exposure.

In the second case, the patient appears misinformed. He may be trying to justify the use of THC for reasons other than relief of pain. In states where THC is legal, this may not be a critical problem. However, the clinician is obligated to inform the patient of the potential side effects and consequences. Even in states where THC is legal, prudence would dictate the use of a proper medical agreement and consent form. The issue of continuing to prescribe opioids is a delicate one. The decision should involve consultation with one's professional board and an awareness of the local standard of care.

KEY POINTS TO REMEMBER

- The use of non-FDA approved therapies is often not covered by malpractice insurance. Before prescribing, the clinician should be sure patients are covered. Traditional malpractice insurance will list any cannabis-related prescriptions or treatments as an exclusion.
- THC is still considered a Schedule I drug by the Drug Enforcement Administration as of June 2020.
- The term "medical" can be misleading. If one successfully uses alcohol at night to induce sleep, does it become "medical alcohol"?
- Absent any appropriate controls and oversite, one cannot fully trust the product labeling and therapeutic claims, even for CBD/hemp.
- In the clinical setting, the benefits must be documented and outweigh the risks.

Further Reading

Aizpurua-Olaizola O, Elezgarai J, Rico-Barrio I, Zaradonna I, Etxebarria N, Usobiaga A. Targeting the endocannabinoid system: future therapeutic strategies. *Drug Disc Today.* 2017;22(1):105–110.

Bisogno T, Hanus L, De Petrocellis L, Tchilibon S, Ponde DE, Brandi I. Molecular targets for cannabidiol and its synthetic analogues: effect on vanilloid VR1 receptors and on the cellular uptake and enzymatic hydrolysis of anandamide. *Br J Pharmacol.* 2001;134:845–852.

Bonn-Miller MO, Loflin MJE, Thomas BF, Marcu JP, Hyke T, Vandrey R. Labeling accuracy of cannabidiol extracts sold online. *JAMA.* 2017;318(17):1708–1709.

Booth JK, Bohlmann J. Terpenes in Cannabis sativa—from plant genome to humans. *Plant Sci.* 2019;284:67–72.

Booth JK, Page JE, Bohlmann J. Terpene synthases from Cannabis sativa. *PLoS One.* 2017;12(3):e0173911. https://doi.org/10.1371/journal.pone.0173911

Carrier EJ, Auchampach JA, Hillard CJ. Inhibition of an equilibrative nucleoside transporter by cannabidiol: a mechanism of cannabinoid immunosuppression. *Proc Natl Acad Sci U S A.* 2006;103(20):7895–7900.

Centers for Disease Control and Prevention. CDC guideline for prescribing opioids for chronic pain—United States. *MMWR Morb Mortal Wkly Rep.* 2016;65(1):1–49. cdc.gov/mmwr/volumes/65/rr/pdfs/rr6501e1.pdf

Controlled Substance Act, 1970. www.dea.gov/controlled-substances-act

Donvito G, Nass S, Wilkerson JL, Curry ZA, Schurman LD, Kinsey SG, Lichtman AH. The endogenous cannabinoid system: a budding source of targets for treating inflammatory and neuropathic pain. *Neuropsychopharmacology.* 2017;43(1):52–79.

Ghasemiesfe M, Barrow B, Leonard S, Keyhani S, Korenstein D. Association between marijuana use and risk of cancer: a systematic review and meta-analysis. *JAMA.* 2019;2(11):e1916318. doi:10.1001/jamanetworkopen.2019.16318

González-Burgos E1, Gómez-Serranillos MP. Terpene compounds in nature: a review of their potential antioxidant activity. *Curr Med Chem.* 2012;19(31):5319–5341.

Greydanus DE, Hawver EK, Greydanus MM, Merrick J. Marijuana: current concepts. *Front Public Health.* 2013;1:42. http://dx.doi.org/10.3389/fpubh.2013.00042

Hazekamp A, Grotenhermen F. Review on clinical studies with cannabis and cannabinoids 2005–2009. *Cannabinoids.* 2010;5:1–21.

Iffland K, Grotenhermen F. An update on safety and side effects of cannabidiol: a review of clinical data and relevant animal studies. *Cannabis Cannabinoid Res.* 2017;2(1):39–154.

Measuring Colorado's "great experiment" with marijuana. *CBS News*; 2018 Jan. 7.

Panche AN, Diwan AD, Chandra SR. Flavonoids: an overview. *J Nutri Sci.* 2017;5(e47):1–15.

Pandey R, Mousawy K, Nagarkatti M, Nagarkatti P. Endocannabinoids and immune regulation. *Pharmacol Res.* 2009;60(2):85–92.

Paul SE, Hatoum AS, Fine JD, et al. Associations between prenatal cannabis exposure and childhood outcomes: results from the ABCD study. *JAMA Psychiatry*. 2020. doi:10.1001/jamapsychiatry.2020.2902

Pertwee RG. Cannabinoid pharmacology: the first 66 years. *Br J Pharmacol*. 2006;147(Suppl 1):S163–S171.

Russo EB, Burnett A, Hall B, Parker KK. Agonistic properties of cannabidiol at 5-HT1a receptors. *Neurochem Res*. 2005;30:1037–1043.

Sturgeon JA, Khan J, Hah JM, Hilmoe H, Hong J, Ware MA, Mackey SC. Clinical profiles of concurrent cannabis use in chronic pain: a CHOIR study. *Pain Med*. 2020;1–8. doi:10.1093/pm/pnaa060

The health effects of cannabis and cannabinoids: the current state of evidence and recommendations for research. Washington, DC: National Academies Press; 2017.

19 Teenager With Disabling Leg Pain

HM is an 18-year-old female referred with severe right leg pain. She had an injury to her foot resulting in an open reduction with internal fixation of the right ankle. She began to show dystrophic symptoms and was diagnosed with complex regional pain syndrome (CRPS). She had a difficult time tolerating physical therapy. However, she did fairly well until she dislocated her kneecap, aggravating the CRPS and resulting in it spreading to her knee. She underwent additional surgery involving a lateral release, relocated patella, and medial collateral ligament. This intensified her neuropathic pain symptoms. She was unable to attend school regularly, but maintained her grades. Her treating pediatric neurologist released her after her 18th birthday. The patient wants to avoid habit-forming substances and does not want to consider neuromodulation. She has received minimal relief from traditional antiepileptic drugs and blocks. She is concerned about graduating high school and being able to attend college. Her bother has a similar problem and is incapacitated by it.

Who do you do now?

BACKGROUND

Clinicians and patients are often encouraged to use complementary and alternative medicine, especially in an effort to minimize or avoid opioids. The terms *complementary* and *alternative* are frequently used together. In fact, they can have very different meanings and implications. Wesa and Cassileth (2009) describe complementary therapies (medicine) as a group of diagnostic and therapeutic disciplines that are often used together with conventional medicine. *Alternative medicine*, on the other hand, is the term for medical products and practices that are not part of standard care and are used in place of it. Indeed, the authors assert that the use of the two terms together

> lends an unwarranted legitimacy to the alternative treatments and taints the value of adjunctive, evidence-based complementary modalities . . . Alternative treatments are unproven or disproved remedies . . . complementary therapies are used in conjunction with mainstream medical therapies and are evidence-based. (p. 1241)

Perhaps one of the most overlooked, underappreciated, and underutilized complementary therapies is nutrition/dietary supplements (ie, functional nutrition; Tennant, 2011). Although frequently ignored, the evidenced-based data supporting the role of nutrition in pain is rather substantial.

In regards to chronic pain, there is a good deal of truth to the statement "We are what we eat." To remain strong and function properly (ie, to be healthy), the peripheral nervous system requires the consistent feeding of oxygen and nutrition through blood flow. Malnutrition, poor circulation, and excessive blood sugar and triglycerides may either disrupt the flow of blood to nerve cells and/or cause blood to be insufficient in essential vitamins and minerals (Tonelli et al, 2009). When nerve cells are deprived, the outer membrane becomes weaker, leaving nerve cells more susceptible to oxidative stress or starvation. The stress signals sent to the central nervous system are interpreted as pain. Often nerve pain is described as sharp, shooting, tingling, or burning. These symptoms are frequently associated with poor nutrition from either excessive carbohydrate or insufficient vitamin/mineral consumption. In a chronic setting, the neuropathic pain process is driven by inflammation and oxidative damage (Schomberg et al,

2012). In an acute setting, similar pain sensations may be driven by consumption of allergens and/or highly inflammatory foods such as processed sugars and oils (Velanta et al, 2015).

ASSESSMENT

There are several ways of assessing potential dietary causes of nerve pain and inflammation. The Australian Healthy Eating Quiz (www.healthyeatingquiz.com.au) is a simple questionnaire based on the criteria established by the diet quality index tool. The Dietary Quality Index (Haines et al, 1999) may not be a meaningful tool for the diagnosis of chronic neuropathic pain diseases; however, when combined with the Malnutrition Screening Tool (Ferguson et al, 1999), these tools can give healthcare providers an idea of whether blood work and allergy testing are an appropriate next step. Patient interview remains the most valuable assessment tool available for determining the necessity and degree of dietary interventions, and initial patient interviews should include discussions of daily diet and activity patterns; family history of diabetes, cardiovascular disease, or mental health disorders; history of weight fluctuations; sleep patterns; and energy levels.

The case of HM is of particular interest and has practical application, as the mother makes direct interview with the patient difficult. In treating patients who live with a caregiver, it may be beneficial to have the caregiver present as that person is often in control of dietary patterns and is a witness to physical activity. However, when an individual is self-reliant, they may be reluctant to be as honest in the presence of partners and/or parents for fear of appearing critical or ungrateful. Nevertheless, interview is the best assessment tool available, and all efforts should be made by healthcare providers to seek honest answers. Questions should be oriented toward dietary patterns, how the patient feels 60 to 90 minutes postprandial, and the patient's sleep patterns and physical activity.

The interview with HM reveals that consumption of poultry meats (eg, chicken and turkey) causes discomfort that the patient describes as allergic reactions. She notes these reactions occur even if poultry is indirectly consumed as a result of cross-contamination, as may occur at restaurants or cafeterias. She admits that she responds well to the consumption of red meat but shows symptoms of biliary dyskinesia and pancreatitis when consuming cuts of red meat that are higher in fat. The reported reactions are not substantiated by allergy testing. Due to the aforementioned dietary restrictions, the patient admits to consuming sugary carbohydrates. She has a tendency to use food as comfort during times of increased stress related to her health concerns. HM's self-reported dietary patterns reveal consumption of food items and quantities that would likely lead to chronic hyperglycemia even in nondiabetics. The overconsumption of highly processed, sugary carbohydrates is consistent with increased symptoms of neuropathy (Torres and Nowson, 2007).

Beyond self-reported food allergies and gastrointestinal complications when consuming higher fat foods, blood work has consistently revealed low serum ferritin but normal red blood cell count. Although the patient has not been previously diagnosed as diabetic or prediabetic, research supports that uncontrolled blood glucose may damage nerve cells, leading to neuropathic pain, and iron deficiencies can impair glucose homeostasis and glycemic control (Soliman et al, 2017). It is critical to note that research supports a positive correlation between CRPS and thyroid function (Schwartzman, 2012; Tennant, 2013), and iron is a critical mineral for proper thyroid function (Soppi, 2015).

In the case of HM, we are left with several important considerations:

- Improve flow of blood and nutrients to peripheral nerves
- Encourage proper liver and gallbladder function to avoid gastric distress
- Provide nutrient-dense food alternatives that would allow HM to avoid allergens and inflammatory fats without turning to highly processed high sugar foods
- Promote healthy caloric intake and activity to manage weight, improve blood flow, and promote hormonal balance

TREATMENT

The most important consideration when implementing a dietary/nutritional intervention is compliance. Because insurance companies rarely offer coverage for dietary supplements, cost is often an issue, as is convenience and personal preference. If the recommended intervention does not fit the patient's lifestyle, budget, or flavor penchant, compliance, and thus a successful outcome, are unlikely. Discussion with patients will reveal what foods and eating schedules best suit their circumstances, and working within these boundaries will increase compliance and improve outcomes. HM is planning to go to a college where living in a dorm room is a Year 1 mandate. She has concerns that the food made available in the cafeteria will spark allergic reactions and gastric distress. Unfortunately, in a cafeteria setting all food is subject to cross-contamination, so avoidance of allergens is not feasible. Additionally, HM has concerns that she will not have access to the comfort foods she tends toward during times of stress but that encourage chronic inflammation.

After discussion with the patient, we agree on minor lifestyle changes and a dietary supplement regimen that includes the following:

- Avoidance of foods that cause allergic reactions including edema
- Replacement of high sugar foods with high antioxidant fruits and vegetables
- Supplementation with Ox Bile and digestive enzymes to detoxify the gallbladder and assist the processing of fats
- Supplementation with milk thistle to protect the liver
- Supplementation with phosphatidylcholine to protect the liver, promote hormonal balance, and improve insulin sensitivity
- Consumption of meal replacement shakes in the form of beef protein isolate that provide balanced nutritional support and highly absorbable haem iron to support thyroid function and improve glucose metabolism

HM is seen in the clinic six months later for a routine follow-up. The patient has lost 20 pounds, and both HM and mother confirm that she was succeeding at college and enjoying a social life. The beef isolate protein shakes allow her to consume calories without avoiding social situations because of gastric distress or consuming high amounts of sugar. The nutrient support has improved her energy levels, which supports class attendance and campus involvement. Over the course of 6 months, HM's medical doctor notes successful discontinuation of tapentadol and tramadol for pain relief and increased involvement in physical therapy.

This case illustrates the how nutritional intervention can significantly contribute to the overall treatment protocol. The psychologist addressed issues with the school, where, despite excellent academic performance, graduation was uncertain secondary to concerns over irregular attendance. In addition, the mother's overprotectiveness and the patient's avoidance behavior were addressed. Physical therapy continued with desensitization and implementation of a home-based exercise program. Medication was kept to a minimum. The addition of functional nutrition accelerated HM's progress and was the one aspect of treatment that addressed the underlying cause of the pain. Furthermore, it provided the patient with the skills and confidence needed to maintain her gains while at college. Her ability to successfully discontinue the use of opioids, secondary to improved pain control, was very gratifying to her and reinforced the importance of nutritionally based lifestyle changes.

KEY POINTS TO REMEMBER

- Patient interview is the most relevant assessment tool.
- Review of dietary trends, activity level, weight fluctuations, and family history of comorbid conditions should be part of any initial evaluation.
- Proper lifestyle management is critical to the control of chronic pain. Patients must avoid high amounts of sugar and processed carbohydrates, practice self-care, and develop skills for managing stress.
- Many dietary supplements have performed comparably to prescription medications in controlled trials. The onus is on healthcare providers to educate themselves on the availability of alternative and adjunct therapies.
- Inflammation is at the root of chronic pain conditions, and many daily choices are either proinflammatory or anti-inflammatory. Identifying and replacing the daily activities that are promoting inflammation are critical components of the care plan.
- While prescription medications can be effective tools for treating chronic pain, patients often view their prescriptions

(or the threat of losing them) as an excuse to continue harmful behaviors.
- Dietary supplements are only as effective as the lifestyle being supplemented; the patient's lifestyle choices are a limiting factor to the effectiveness of medications.

Further Reading

Ferguson M, Capra S, Bauer J, Banks M. Development of a valid and reliable malnutrition screening tool for adult acute hospital patients. *Nutrition*. 1999;15:458–464.

Haines PS, Siega-Riz AM, Popkin BM. The Diet Quality Index Revised: a measurement instrument for populations. *J Am Diet Assoc*. 1999;99(6):697–704.

Schomberg D, Ahmed M, Miranpuri G, Olson J, Resnick DK. Neuropathic pain: role of inflammation, immune response, and ion channel activity in central injury mechanisms. *Ann Neurosci*. 2012;19(3):25–32.

Schwartzman RJ. Systemic complications of complex regional pain syndrome. *Neurosci Med*. 2012;1-18.

Soliman AS, De Sanctis V, Yassin M, Soliman N. Iron deficiency anemia and glucose metabolism. *Acta Biomed*. 2017;88(1):112–118.

Soppi E. Iron deficiency is the main cause of symptom persistence in patients treated for hypothyroidism. *Thyroid*. 2015;25(suppl 1):A-74.

Tennant F. A diet for patients with chronic pain. *Pract Pain Manag*. 2011;6:1–6.

Tennant F. The physiologic effects of pain on the endocrine system. *Pain Ther*. 2013;2:75–86.

Tonelli M, Wiebe N, Hemmelgarn B, Klarenbach S, Field K, Manns B, Thadhani R, Gill J. Trace elements in hemodialysis patients: a systematic review and meta-analysis. *BMC Med*. 2009;7:1–12.

Torres SJ, Nowson CA. Relationship between stress, eating behavior, and obesity. *Nutrition*. 2007;23 (11–12):887–889.

Valenta R, Hochwallner H, Linhart B, Pahr S. Food allergies: the basics. *Gastroenterology*. 2015;148(6):1120–1131.

Wesa K, Cassileth NR. Is there a role for complementary therapy in the management of leukemia? *Expert Rev Anticancer Ther*. 2009;9:1241–1249.

General Considerations

20 Psychogenic Pain: A Useful Concept?

Pain can also be fully internally generated instead of driven by afferent input.
— *Grunel and Tolle (2005, pp. 91–92)*

I'm suffering in my mind because I can't suffer in my body.
— *Namo, a leprosy patient, quoted in Brand and Yancey (1997, p. 125)*

INTRODUCTION

Psychogenic or psychogenesis is defined in Webster's dictionary as "an event that originates or develops within the psyche/mind; the development of a physical disorder resulting from mental conflict versus organic cause." The ambiguity of this term is enhanced by the psyche being declared as an entity beyond natural or known physical processes, apparently sensitive to forces beyond the physical world. The notion of psychogenic pain got a good deal of traction with Engel (1959). Indeed, he proposed the existence of pain-prone personality. As recently as 2008, Italian neurosurgeon Giovanni Broggi asserted that human pain could be divided into two main categories: physical pain and psychological pain. He went on to describe one as "clearly physical, the other having more to deal with the mind" (p. 901).

Ones understanding of the term "psychogenic pain" can significantly influence the approach to the assessment and treatment of chronic pain. The purpose of this chapter is to provide (i) a brief history of the term psychogenic, (ii) a brief review of some the factors that can influence the development and maintenance of chronic pain, (iii) alternative frameworks within which to understand chronic pain, and (iv) recommendations regarding the disposition of the term "psychogenic." Essentially, it is an attempt to disentangle the concept of psychogenic pain and the continued tendency, intentional or not, to sustain the dichotomy of psychogenic versus somatogenic pain, the latter being considered to be "real" pain.

At times, perhaps more often than not, the precise factor(s) contributing to the development and maintenance of chronic pain may not be fully appreciated because of the sophistication and complexity of the assessment required to do so. In addition, the human body and brain are complex adaptive systems. That is, the factor(s) of greatest influence at one point in time can, and do, change with circumstances. This ever-changing land-scape is fertile ground for unfounded speculations regarding the etiology of chronic pain.

HISTORY OF THE TERM "PSYCHOGENIC PAIN"

The contemporary use of the term "psychogenic pain" has its roots in psy-chodynamically dominated theory. Pain was viewed as a central part of psychic development and function. It involved human relationships and punishment occurring early in one's developmental history. Pain came to be associated with aggression, power in childhood, the actual or imagined loss of a loved one, and feelings of a sexual nature. Psychogenic pain was most likely to occur (i) when external circumstances failed to satisfy the un-conscious need to suffer; (ii) as a response to real, imagined, or fantasized loss; or (iii) in response to guilt evoked by intense aggressive or forbidden sexual feelings.

During the time of Sigmund Freud (b. 1856–d. 1939), there was a change in the way the brain and mind were conceptualized. The psyche became the mediator between the brain and the mind. It evaluated and interpreted events to which the individual was exposed, especially those occurring early in life. The psyche included the superego, ego, and id. This psychiatric triumvirate ultimately determined the manner in which the individual responded to life events. Much of this processing of events occurred outside the individual's awareness (ie, at the unconscious level). The patient's personality and manner in which he or she dealt with life was thought to be established by adolescence.

In 1917 Raether claimed that if a deviation in functioning existed (eg, low-back pain), it must have a physical cause (Raether, 1917, as cited in Lutz et al, 2003). If an anatomical abnormality could not be found, he declared that the technology was simply not sophisticated enough to find it. Once found, the abnormality was to be addressed surgically. If the data from the physical examination and diagnostic testing did not add up, the problem was declared to be psychogenic and beyond the reach of acceptable medical therapies. In this regard, Raether observed, "Even non-specialists know from experience during the war and the numerous publications about 'war-neurotics,' that the psychogenic component is far more important than anyone would have expected" (cited in Lutz et al, 2003, p. 1902).

Psychogenic causes of pain were alluded to in nearly 60% of articles published from 1900 to 1950. Some of the proposed psychogenic explanations for chronic pain included sexual neurasthenia, excessive masturbation, abnormal and exaggerated sexuality, fears, and unfulfilled wishes. However, the trend all but disappeared in the 1970s. But there was a resurgence between 1980 and 2000. This pattern seemed to parallel the advent of more sophisticated imaging technology and improved surgical outcomes. That is, the more that could be seen, and the better the surgical outcomes were thought to be, the less emphasis was placed on psychogenic causes. More recently, the term "psychogenic" was replaced by "medically unexplained symptoms" (MUS). The phrase appears in both the third (DSM-III; American Psychiatric Association [APA], 1988) and fourth (DSM-IV; APA, 1995) editions of the *Diagnostic and Statistical Manual of Mental Disorders*. It was intended to reflect the imprecision and uncertainty of a diagnosis and to hopefully avoid stigmatizing the patient.

In the DSM-IV (APA, 1995), the term "psychogenic pain" was replaced with "pain disorder." The diagnosis of pain disorder was considered appropriate when psychological factors were judged to play a significant role in the onset, severity, exacerbation, or maintenance of pain. This effectively eliminated the process of a diagnosis by exclusion. This appeared to be a shift away from appealing to the unconscious processes proposed by Freud to the more conventional and observable psychological factors. Unfortunately, the tendency to describe pain as psychogenic when a clear physical cause cannot be identified remains.

The International Association for the Study of Pain (IASP) has been endowed with the responsibility of developing a nomenclature and classification system for pain. The second edition of the *Classification of Chronic Pain* (Merskey and Bogduk, 1994) uses the phrase "pain of psychological origin." There are three main categories: (i) delusional/hallucinatory; (ii) hysterical, conversion, or hypochondriacal; and (iii) associated with depression. For the diagnosis of pain be properly applied, there needs to be evidence of pain without an adequate pathophysiological explanation (diagnosis by exclusion). However, there must also be separate evidence to support the view that a psychiatric illness is present. Proof of the presence of psychological factors by (i) relationship in time or (ii) the patient avoiding undesirable activity or obtaining support from the environment otherwise not forthcoming (Merskey and Bogduk, 1994, p. 55) is required.

The IASP definition of pain as "an unpleasant sensory and emotional experience associated with actual or potential tissue damage, or described in terms of such damage" allows for the experience of pain to occur in the absence of any external noxious stimulation or activation of the nociceptive system by a peripheral stimulus. Indeed, Melzack (1989) suggested that a physical body was not necessary to experience pain. The implication being that it can be generated by the brain. However, modern pain medicine encompasses a number of procedures and techniques designed to identify the presumed pain generator.

The term "psychogenic pain" tends to be applied when this so called pain generator cannot be found, thus a diagnosis by exclusion. However, several lines of evidence call into question this notion of a pain generator. First, it is well known that 30% to 40% of individuals with abnormal imaging studies have no complaints of pain (Jensen et al, 1994). Second, positive discograms (anatomically abnormal disc) have been found in asymptomatic patients (Carragee et al, 1999, 2000). Third, epidural scarring thought to be the cause of continuing pain after surgery is not always associated with pain. Finally, there are multiple chemical mediators (eg, substance P and glutamate) and nociceptive processing changes (ie, central sensitization) associated with pain that can be independent of any identified structural abnormality. These observations suggest that physical damage and pain are not the same. Indeed, Merskey and Bogduk (1994) stated that "activity induced in the nociceptor and the nociceptive pathways by a noxious stimulus is not pain, which is always a psychological state even though we may well appreciate that pain most often has an approximate physical cause" (p. 210). As will be outlined later in this chapter, there are many subtle factors that influence the experience of pain that may not be readily observed or measured.

MODELS OF PAIN PROCESSING

The phrase "pain processing" refers to the interaction of the various peripheral and central mechanism involved in generating the experience of pain. There are several models of pain processing that attempt to explain the presence of chronic pain in the absence of what Tracey (2005) refers to as a nociceptive drive and when the pain is not improved by pharmacological or surgical therapy or altered by natural disease progression. Tracey listed four options: (i) unidentified remnants of the nociceptive drive or tissue damage, (ii) emotional or cognitive elements within the brain, (iii) amplification or alteration of nociceptive or nonnociceptive input due to sensitization within the nervous system, or (iv) the patient's imagination.

Melzack and Casey (1968) described pain processing as involving three principle components. The sensory/discriminative component informs the person of the precise location and quality of their pain. The affective/motivational component reflects the impact of emotional states such as depression, anxiety, and fear. The parts of the brain associated with this component also serve as a repository for many repressed and past emotional traumas—the emotional aspect of which can be activated by new physical or emotional trauma and thus impact the degree of pain and suffering experienced by the patient. Finally, the cognitive/evaluative component is the harbinger of our knowledge, expectations, and meaning as it relates to the injury and subsequent pain. The effect of self-fulfilling prophecies such as "You'll never get any better" and "You will be in a wheelchair in 10 years" in a sense reside here and become manifest in the presence of physical harm by enhancing or turning up the volume, as it were, on the output of the interactive effects of the sensory and affective components.

Price (1999, 2000) outlined a pain processing system containing four components: (i) nociception, (ii) primary pain affect, (iii) secondary pain affect, and (iv) the behavioral response. In his model, nociceptive activity triggered by some event is transmitted to the sensory component of the brain. If this event is perceived by the person as intrusive or threatening in some way, it is immediately followed by pain unpleasantness (eg, distress, fear, annoyance). This pain unpleasantness gives way to second-order appraisals such as interruption in activities, difficulty enduring pain, or concern for the future. Extended pain affect (depression, frustration, anxiety, anger) then follows. Finally, there is a behavioral response (avoidance, withdrawal, relief-seeking).

The models proposed by Melzack and Casey (1968) and Price (1999, 2000) clearly state that what is ultimately felt as pain is the product of a complex and dynamic interaction of multiple components and systems and may well be disproportionate to the inciting event. If these models of pain processing are correct, then, by extension, any increase or decrease in negative emotions or maladaptive cognitive states should alter the pain (McCracken et al, 1998). Thus, the basis for cognitively oriented therapies.

THE CONTEXTUAL BASIS OF PAIN

The term "context" relates to the circumstances that form the setting for an event, statement, or idea and allows for a great understanding of it. The qualitative and qualitative aspects of chronic pain are determined by many factors: its context. This section reviews a variety of these factors and the means by which they can influence the experience of pain.

Words and Pain Rating

A patient's numerical pain rating, generally obtained using a 0–10 scale, is often used to judge the severity or intensity of pain. Yet, the numerical pain rating can be influenced by a number of environmental factors including perceived consequences, mood, gender of the clinician, and presence of a reinforcing spouse. Even the use of certain language to describe a potentially painful stimulus can influence the report of pain and its intensity. For example, the use of the term "pain" in place of "cold sensation" (Lang et al, 2005) or "You will feel a bee sting" in place of "It will numb the area" (Varelmann et al, 2010) has been shown to increase the reported intensity of pain.

Depression

Psychological factors, such as mood, have been known to influence pain affect and intensity. The association of depression and pain has been well recognized. Indeed, it has been estimated that up to 65% of clinically depressed patients have unexplained pain, and 37% (range 5%–85% depending on which study is quoted) of patients with chronic pain manifest clinically significant depression. The more the pain is allowed to interfere with daily functions, the greater the depressive symptoms. This may be a reflection of Ferster's (1973) reinforcement theory of depression. This theory hypothesized that depression is associated with the degree of rewarding events the person engages in and the amount of positive reinforcement from others. Therefore, as the individual with pain avoids engaging in desirable activities such as work, sporting events, family interactions, religious services, and sexual intimacy, etc., depression begins and worsens, intensifying the overall experience of pain. Therapies that emphasize a return to activity or the development of new reinforcing activities are more likely to affect depression and pain. Treatments that reduce pain without improving the frequency of rewarding activity may not be as successful at improving mood.

Expectation
Expectations of a painful stimulus are known to amplify perceived unpleasantness of even innocuous stimulation, but they appear to have little effect on the reported pain intensity. In other words, when a person knows they will be exposed to a variety of events, some of which will be painful and others not, but without any means of knowing exactly when the painful ones will occur, even the previously nonpainful events will be experienced as painful. Yet, when asked to rate the degree of perceived unpleasantness and intensity of the event, the intensity rating remains unchanged, but the unpleasantness rating is higher. In essence, it is the brain's affective/emotional response to the stimuli that is influenced, not the intensity of the sensation. Likewise, a startle response is substantially altered when the event is predictable and expected compared to when it is not (Sawamoto et al, 2000).

Pain Catastrophizing
In clinical practice, it is not uncommon to encounter patients reporting incessant ruminations regarding their pain (ie, pain catastrophizing [PC]). They worry that the pain will never get better and obsess over their feelings

of helplessness. Descriptions of their pain and its effects on their life tend to be very exaggerated and dramatic. Such patients, and their complaints, are often dismissed and disregarded. They are frequently referred for psychological or psychiatric therapy, based on the clinician's belief that pain, if it exists at all, is imaged or psychogenic.

One study (Gracely et al, 2004) examined a group of patients diagnosed with fibromyalgia and demonstrating high levels of PC using functional magnetic resonance imaging (fMRI) neuroimaging. They discovered increased activity in areas of the brain related to anticipation of pain, attention to pain, emotional aspects of pain, and motor control. It seemed that PC influenced pain perception through altering attention and anticipation and increasing the emotional response to pain. What was not apparent was whether this pattern of brain activity was (i) somehow genetically determined, (ii) linked to certain types of personalities, (iii) a result of early childhood rearing practices, (iv) current patterns of reinforcement, or (v) a combination of these factors.

Suggestibility

Derbyshire et al (2003, 2004) examined eight highly hypnotizable subjects exposed to a thermal stimulus while undergoing fMRI scanning. A single tap on the hand announced the arrival of the painful heat stimulus, while two taps signified a rest period. Although there was a total of six trials, the painful heat stimulus was presented on only three of the six trials. Under hypnosis, the subjects were told to imagine the painful heat stimulus (hypnotic-induced hallucination). Hallucinatory pain occurred on the trials when no stimulus was presented and appeared to involve the same brain structures as those activated by the actual stimulus. Consistent with the findings of Raij et al (2005) using suggestion-prone individuals, the researchers concluded that events often *feel* real or unreal rather than are known to be real or unreal. That is, pain stimulated by a mechanism other than peripheral noxious stimulation may well feel the same to the patient.

Early Life Stress/Anxiety

Visceral pain involves internal organs, including the bowel, bladder, and stomach. Irritable bowel syndrome, chronic stomach upset (dyspepsia), and noncardiac chest pain have often been considered to be a result of anxiety.

Human (Myers and Greenwood-Van Meerveld, 2009) and animal (Larauche et al, 2011) studies have shown that early life stresses created by such events as maternal separation can result in an increased visceromotor response to colorectal distention or visceral hyperalgesia. Therefore, patients may complain of pain even in presence of normal visceral activity. Unfortunately, such complaints often lead to repeated invasive investigations and surgery, the outcome of which is to cause further irritation and the creation of adhesions. While it is clear that anxiety and stress play a role in the development of such disorders, there is also an underlying physiological mechanism that should discourage interpreting disorders as a purely psychological phenomenon.

The lack of any significant improvement in pain following spine surgery undertaken primarily as a treatment for chronic pain has been used as evidence that the pain is driven by psychological rather than physical variables. However, Schofferman et al (1992) determined that many of the patients who failed to improve had been exposure to one or more *developmental traumas*, including physical or sexual abuse, evidence of alcohol and or drug abuse in a primary caregiver, being abandoned by a primary caregiver, or emotional neglect or abuse. Prevalence of abuse in women referred to multidisciplinary pain centers is approximately 48%. (Drossman et al, 1995; Green et al, 1999; Wurtele et al, 1990). Brain imaging studies have identified a reduction in the size of the hippocampus (Bremner et al, 1997; Stein et al, 1997) and higher levels of cortisol (Weissbeckera et al, 2006) in adult women with a history of childhood sexual abuse. These data suggest that such event can be associated with anatomical and hormonal consequence that could persist.

Patients with a history of trauma tend to have more sites of pain, higher pain intensities, greater use of healthcare system, and greater drug and alcohol abuse. More likely to report gastrointestinal, pelvic, fibromyalgia, and head pain. They frequently consider themselves victims and powerless rather than as an empowered survivor. A history of developmental trauma is considered to be a potential risk factor for a poor outcome from interventional and surgical procedures. It is unclear why some persons with histories of abuse respond like those without such a history. Taken as a whole, the data clearly suggest that childhood trauma can influence the degree of the pain response in adult life may well have physiological correlates.

Conditioning and Learning

Another means by which pain can be experienced without peripheral stimulation is through conditioning and learning. Flor et al (1997) demonstrated increased in pain-related electrical brain wave activity in response to a colored light after the light had been associated with previously associated with a painful shock to the finger. Similarly, this type of *conditioned nociception* was found to occur in the monkey (Duncan et al, 1987) after a light had been repeatedly used to signal the onset of potential painful stimulus. In this instance, recordings were made from the spinal thalamic tract, which is known to be the nociceptive transmission system conducting impulses from the periphery to the brain.

There is strong evidence that patients receiving a good deal of positive or negative reinforcement for their pain behavior may experience more pain and pain-related disability than those who do not. Indeed, when patients with chronic low back pain were given a mild electrical shock to their back in the presence of an overly sympathetic spouse, enhanced activity in the brain's pain matrix was noted compared to when the spouse was absent or if the patient's spouse tended to be more apathetic (Flor et al, 1987). Observations of this type have helped to form the basis for pain therapies that incorporate learning theory and conditioning principles.

Epigenetics

Genetics has been found to account for up to 50% of some pain conditions (Fillingim et al, 2008; Mogil, 1999). Epigenetics (EMGEX) is a related but different phenomenon. EMGEX (Zhang and Meaney, 2010) describes heritable changes in gene expression that do not involve DNA mutation. These changes can be a result of any number of stresses. For example, higher levels of cortisol and a greater likelihood of developing posttraumatic stress syndrome have been found in the offspring of Holocaust survivors and American women who were pregnant during the 9/11 World Trade Center attacks (Yehuda et al, 2002, 2005). Genetic polymorphisms that affect stress responsiveness include variations in catechol-o-methyltransferase, serotonin transporter, and alpha 2-adrenergic receptor genes. Offspring of pregnant women carrying these polymorphisms may acquire an overly responsive stress-response system as a consequence of being exposed to the by-products of the mother's enhanced stress response.

Offspring of parents with a history of chronic pain demonstrated enhanced pain sensitivity potentially attributable to alternation in endogenous opioid functions (Bruehl and Chung, 2006). There is evidence showing an alteration in gene expression in pregnant women genetically predisposed to being more sensitive to stress when exposed to certain types of stress (Buffington, 2009). The consequences of EMGEX, such as neuroendocrine abnormalities, are passed on to the offspring. One model demonstrates how heightened sensitivity and vulnerability to stress and the development of disorders as chronic pelvic pain, chronic fatigue syndrome, irritable bowel syndrome, interstitial cystitis, and fibromyalgia can result from an epigenetic modulation of gene expression (EMGEX; McGowan et al, 2009).

This altered genetic pattern is passed on to the offspring, rendering them genetically vulnerable and predisposed to developing certain types of disorders or symptoms in response to what might otherwise be considered normal stresses. However, there are a number of studies suggesting the presence of critical developmental periods when offspring are more vulnerable (Buffington, 2006). It is also during this time period that high levels of physical contact and maternal responsiveness may mitigate a genetic predisposition toward a more extreme stress reaction (Anisman et al, 1998; deKloet et al, 1996). These observations represent yet another example of the complex adaptive nature of the human organism (system).

Immune System

Glial cells are nonneuronal cells that maintain homeostasis for neurons in the central and peripheral nervous systems. These cells serve five functions: (i) surround neurons and hold them in place, (ii) supply nutrient and oxygen to neurons, (iii) insulate one neuron from another, (iv) destroy pathogens and remove dead neurons, and (v) assist neurons in forming synaptic connections. Abnormal glial cell functioning can sensitize nociceptive neurons and cause the release of pronociceptive cytokines and neurotrophins. These pro-inflammatory substances have been linked to the onset and maintenance of chronic pain. Indeed, anti-inflammatory factors like interleukin (IL)-10, IL-4, IL-1 alpha, and transforming growth factor-beta 1 are being investigated as treatment of neuropathic pain (Mike et al, 2013). Some have suggested that chronic pain may be a result of gliopathy, or dysregulation of glial functions in the central nervous system and protracted abstinence syndrome (Jia et al, 2013).

Activation of the innate immune system by some pathogen-associated molecule can also results in the synthesis and release of pro-inflammatory cytokines, including tumor necrosis factor alpha and ILs. The role of IL-1, tumor necrosis factor, and nerve growth factor in pain and being sick has been detailed by Watkins and Maier (2000). One study compared fibromyalgia patients with nonpain controls and found increased levels of IL-6 and IL-8 in the fibromyalgia group. IL-6 is associated with hyperalgesia, fatigue, and depression; IL-8 is associated with sympathetic related pain (Wallace et al, 2001).

The brain cytokine system can undergo sensitization as a result of stimulation during the early stages of development, repeated activation by exposure to environmental stressors, and prior activations by exposure to environmental stressors (Dantzer, 2005). This, in turn, can result in triggering a sickness response consisting of fever, neuroendocrine responses, sickness behavior, and affective and cognitive alterations. Dantzer asserted that somatization "might be nothing else than the outward manifestation of sensitization of the brain cytokine system that is normally activated in response to activation of the innate immune system and mediates the subjective, behavioral and physiological components of sickness" (p. 948).

Brain Morphology

One study (Mansour et al, 2013) examined serial fMRIs of the brain of a group of patients with acute pain. The pain resolved in several of these patients while others developed chronic pain. Within two months, differences in the structure and integrity of the white matter distinguished those whose pain persisted from those where the pain began to resolve. At 12 months, structural differences distinguished patients whose pain resolved versus those that persisted (became chronic). Compared to healthy controls and those whose pain resolved, the white matter in the subjects whose pain became chronic exhibited 30 to 50 years of additional aging. This implicated abnormal brain morphology as a risk factor for the development of chronic pain.

Medically Unexplained Symptoms

The term "medically unexplained (or functional) symptoms" refers to physical symptoms that prompt the sufferer to seek health care but remain unexplained after an appropriate medical evaluation (Richardson and Engel, 2004). Pain second to MUS has often been used synonymously with psychogenic, somatoform, psychological, psychiatric, or imaginary pain. These terms imply that the pain is essentially in the mind of the patient rather associated with some physical abnormality. This is true even in the presence of physical manifestations such as swelling, fever, or muscular abnormalities. Common features of patients identified as having MUS are listed in Box 20.1.

The fifth edition of the *Diagnostic and Statistical Manual of Mental Disorders* (DSM-5; APA, 2013) eliminated the diagnoses of somatization, hypochondriasis, pain disorder, and undifferentiated somatoform disorder, previously subsumed under somatoform disorders. This category was replaced by complex somatic symptom disorder. Furthermore, the phrase 'medically unexplained symptom' was abolished. The diagnosis of somatic symptom disorder is now based on positive (identifiable) cognitive and behavioral features. It may be noteworthy that, when surveyed, even healthy individuals found the term "medically unexplained symptoms" unacceptable (Marks and Hunter, 2015).

According to Dimsdale and Creed (2009), somatic symptoms are one aspect of a complex somatic symptoms disorder. Other aspects include misattributions, excessive concern or preoccupation with symptoms and illness, and increased healthcare utilization. The emphasis is on identifying

---

BOX 20.1   **Common Features of MUS**

- Female
- Early adverse experience
- Sudden onset, often associated with some type of injury or infection
- Multiple coexisting symptoms in the same patient with no set order of onset
- Waxing and waning of symptoms,
- Heightened stress response involving altered adrenocortical and sympathetic nervous system functioning
- Recalcitrance to common treatments

common features versus a diagnosis by exclusion. Somatic symptoms will now be viewed in the context of their severity and intensity as multiple or single, localized or nonspecific.

This change is in line with a more general concerns over terms like "mental illness." It begins to recognize that it may be the pain and not the patient that is abnormal. One can easily imagine that there are times when a strong emotional reaction to pain and its devastating consequences would be considered normal versus some type of mental illness or disorder. Indeed, even within psychiatry, the definition and meaningfulness of the concept of mental illness remains unsettled (Schramme, 2013). A. J. Frances, chairperson of the committee that framed DSM-IV and a contributor to DSM-5, stated, "There could arguably not be a worse term than 'mental disorders' to describe the conditions classified in DSM-IV.' Mental' implies a mind–body dichotomy that is becoming increasingly outmoded" (Frances, 1994, p. viii). Stein et al (2010) have also asserted that the term "mental" (psychogenic) promotes a Cartesian mind–body dualism that is inconsistent with contemporary philosophical and neuroscientific views.

SUMMARY

Several conclusions can be drawn from the previous discussion. First, a person can experience pain in the absence of any stimulation of the peripheral nociceptive system. Second, stimulation of the nociceptive system by a nonnoxious stimulus can be experienced as pain as a result of the impact of psychological factors. Third, painful stimuli can be made more unpleasant without influencing its perceived intensity. Fourth, to the extent that psychogenic pain means pain without stimulation of the peripheral nociceptive system, it does, in fact, exist. Finally, there is the intended, or unintended, consequence of applying a label indicative of a mental illness to a situation in which none may exist.

There can be little doubt as to the presence of a neurophysiological correlates of what is commonly referred to as psychogenic pain. Anticipation and expectation of pain activates the primary somatosensory cortex, anterior cingulate cortex, periaqueductal gray matter, insular cortex, prefrontal cortex, and cerebellum. The use of priming events is associated with increased electroencephalographic activity. Negative emotional states enhance pain perception through involvement of anterior cingulate cortex and insular cortex. Hypnotic suggestion altered pain-evoked activity that was region-specific based on the nature of the suggestion. In addition, the context in which chronic pain exists contains a myriad of environmental, developmental, hormonal, and immune system factors.

Based on these observations, there appears to be several possible types of psychogenic pain. In one type, pain functions as a defense mechanism reflecting some unconscious process, à la Sigmund Freud's notion of a conversion reaction. A second type could be a psychophysiological response in which the pain is mediated by a physiological response (eg, an autonomic or muscular response) to an event. The classical tension headache in response to muscular tightness created in response to stress is an example. A third type of psychogenic pain could be a product of some psychological procedure or process, such as hypnosis or suggestion. Finally, the qualitative and quantitative aspect of pain can be influenced by psychosocial factors, including mood, attention, distraction, and developmental traumas.

However, it may be instructive to recall the IASP's (1976) note on the definition of pain:

> Many people report pain in the absence of tissue damage or any likely pathophysiological cause; usually this happens for psychological reasons. There is usually no way to distinguish their experience from that due to tissue damage if we take the subjective report. If they regard their experience as pain and if they report it in the same ways as pain caused by tissue damage, it should be accepted as pain. (p. 247)

This clearly acknowledges the influential role of psychological factors as regards the *report* of pain versus the pain as being psychological (psychogenic). Furthermore, Merskey (1994), one of the architects of the original IASP definition of pain, makes the point:

> It was evident that patients with psychological distress had experiences of pain in the body which resembled our experiences with physical illness, and both types of experience had to be regarded as pain, despite the lack of a physical cause for some of the former" (p. S75)

This statement appears to further remove any legitimacy from the psychogenic versus real pain distinction. Indeed, Cohen et al (2018) describe psychogenic pain as a "clinically untenable concept" (p. 3).

The argument herein is that there are many pathophysiological process (eg, immune system dysfunction, EMGX, central sensitization, cortical reorganization, microglial activation, etc.) that could easily account for the chronic pain, absent the more obvious and easily discernable anatomical pathology (actual or potential tissues damage; "Pain Terms," 1979). Perhaps it is best to consider any deviation for normal physiological processing on par with structural abnormalities. Unfortunately, the tendency to hold the patient accountable for the shortcomings of medical technology (recognized by Raether 100 years ago) remains. Some (Aydede and Shriver, 2018) have now suggested the terms "nociplastic" or "nocipathic" to capture such situations. Nociplastic pain is defined as "pain that arises from altered nociception despite no clear evidence of actual or threatened tissue damage causing the activation of peripheral nociceptors or evidence for disease or lesion of the somatosensory system causing the pain" (Aydede and Shriver, 2018, p. 1176). Potential etiological factors include immune system dysfunction, microglial activation, EMGEX, central sensitization, and/or cortical reorganization. Fibromyalgia, irritable bowel syndrome, chronic fatigue syndrome, and interstitial cystitis are given as example of diagnostic entities that might be assumed under the term "nociplastic."

Psychogenic, neurotic, nonorganic, and functional pain have been viewed as synonymous. At the heart of the matter is the mind–body problem (Bracken and Thomas, 2002) and the acknowledged uncertainty of the etiology of many pain experiences. Because of the fundamental issues of causality, dualism, and normality, almost 50 years ago Lewis (1972) suggested that the term "psychogenic" be given a decent burial. This sentiment was echoed some 30 years later by Katon et al (2001) when they declared that both disease and distress are capable of producing physical symptoms. It is not productive, they suggested, to dichotomize symptoms as "somatogenic" or "psychogenic" because physiological and psychological processes are involved in all symptom production and perception. Rule-out diagnostic strategies that search for either a medical or a psychiatric cause of a physical symptom are not supported by epidemiological findings indicating a high rate of medical and psychiatric comorbidity. (p. 922).

Hopefully, the elimination of "psychogenic" from the lexicon would lessen some of the fruitless controversies it has elicited including organic versus functional, real versus psychological, and real versus imagined and further remove the discussion from the realm of the metaphysical.

Therefore, it is recommended that the term "psychogenic pain" be abandoned. It continues to be applied as a diagnosis by exclusion. Also, the term suggests that the pain, especially chronic pain, can be something other than "real" pain, and the veracity of patients labeled as manifesting psychogenic pain is repeatedly questioned. Instead, the emphasis should be on identifying (i) historical and predisposing factors that, via epigenetic or other processes, alter the system in such a fashion as to make the emergence of chronic pain more likely; (ii) current psychological and behavioral variables that mediate the severity of the chronic pain, and (iii) factors that influence the homeostatic function of the human complex-adaptive system and, as such, would represent meaningful therapeutic targets. This approach eliminates the issue of mental illness and provides a more rational basis for the development of a treatment algorithm.

Further Reading

American Psychiatric Association. *Diagnostic and Statistical Manual of Mental Disorders.* 3rd ed. rev. Washington, DC: American Psychiatric Association; 1988.

American Psychiatric Association. *Diagnostic and Statistical Manual of Mental Disorders.* 4th ed. Washington, DC: American Psychiatric Association; 1995.

American Psychiatric Association. *Diagnostic and Statistical Manual of Mental Disorders.* 5th ed. Washington, DC: American Psychiatric Association; 2013.

Anisman H, Zaharia MD, Meaney MJ, Merali Z. Do early-life events permanently alter behavioral and hormonal responses to stressors? *Int J Dev Neurosci.* 1998;16(3–4):149–164.

Aydede M, Shriver A. Recently introduced definition of "nociplastic *pain*" by the International Association for the Study of Pain needs better formulation. *Pain.* 2018;159(6):1176–1177.

Bracken TP. Time to move beyond the mind–body split. *BMJ.* 2002;325:1433–1434.

Bremner LD, Randall P, Vermetten E, et al. Magnetic resonance imaging-based measurement of hippocampal volume in posttraumatic stress disorder related to childhood physical and sexual abuse: a preliminary report. *Biol Psychiatry.* 1997;41(1):23–32.

Broggi G. Pain and psychoaffective disorders. *Neurosurgery.* 2008;62(6 Suppl 3):1–19.

Bruehl S, Chung OY. Parental history of chronic *pain* may be associated with impairments in endogenous opioid analgesic systems. *Pain.* 2006;124:287–294.

Buffington CAT. Developmental influences on medically unexplained symptom. *Psychother Psychosom.* 2009;78:139–144.

Carragee EJ, Tanner CM, Khurana S, et al. The rates of false-positive lumbar discography in select patients without low back symptoms. *Spine.* 2000;25:1373–1380.

Carragee EJ, Tanner CM, Yang B, Brito JL, Truong T. False-positive findings on lumbar discography: reliability of subjective concordance assessment during provocative disc injection. *Spine.* 1999;24:2542–2547.

Cohen M, Quintner J, van Rysewyk S. Reconsidering the International Association for the Study of Pain definition of pain. *Pain Rep.* 2018;3(2):e634.

Dantzer R. Somatization: a psychoneuroimmune perspective. *Psychoneuroimmunology.* 2005;30:947–952.

de Kloet ER, Rots NY, Cools AR. Brain–corticosteroid hormone dialogue: slow and persistent. *Cell Mol Neurobiol (Netherlands).* 1996;16(3):345–356.

Derbyshire SW, Whalley M, Oaklet D. Subjects hallucinating pain in the absence of a stimulus activate anterior cingulated, anterior insula, prefrontal and parietal cortices. *J Pain.* 2003;4(2 Suppl):Abstract 754.

Derbyshire SW, Whalley MG, Stenger VA. Oakley DA. Cerebral activation during hypnotically induced and imagined pain. *Neuroimage.* 2004;23:392–401.

Dimsdale J, Creed F. The proposed diagnosis of somatic symptom disorders in DSM-V to replace somatoform disorders in DSM-IV: a preliminary report. *Psychosom Res.* 2009;66(6):473–476.

Drossman DA, Leserman J, Nachman G, et al. Sexual and physical abuse in women with functional or organic gastrointestinal disorders. *Ann Intern Med.* 1990;113:828–833.

Duncan GH, Bushnell MC, Bates R, Dubner R. Task-related responses of monkey medullary dorsal horn neurons. *J Neurophysiol.* 1987;57:289–310.

Engle, GL. Psychogenic pain and the pain prone personality. *Am J Med.* 1959:26;899–918.

Ferster CB. A functional analysis of depression. *Am Psychol.* 1973;28(10):857–879.

Fillingim RB, Wallace MR, Herbstman DM, Ribeiro-Dasilva M, Staud R. Genetic contributions to pain: a review of findings in humans *Oral Dis.* 2008;14(8):673–682.

Flor H, Braun C, Elbert T, Birbaumer N. Extensive reorganization of primary somatosensory cortex in chronic back pain patients. *Neurosci Lett.* 1997;224(1)5–8.

Flor H, Kerns RD, Turk DC. The role of spouse reinforcement, perceived pain, and activity levels of chronic pain patients. *J Psychosom Res.* 1987;31:251–259.

Frances AJ. Foreword. In: Frances A, First MB, Widiger TA, et al, eds. *Philosophical Perspectives on Psychiatric Diagnostic Classification*. Baltimore, MD: Johns Hopkins University Press; 1994:vii–ix.

Gracely RH, Geisser ME, Giesecke T, Grant MA, Williams DA, Clauw DJ. Pain catastrophizing and neural responses to pain among persons with fibromyalgia. *Brain*. 2004;127:835–843.

Green CR, Flowe-Valencia H, Rosenblum L, Tait AR. Do physical and sexual abuse differentially affect chronic pain states in women? *J Pain Symptom Manage*. 1999;18:420–426.

Grunel H, Tolle TR. How physical pain may interact with psychological pain: evidence of a mutual neurobiological basis of emotions and pain. In: Carr D, Loeser JD, Morris DB, eds. *Narrative Pain and Suffering*. Seattle, Washington: IASP Press; 2005:87–112.

Jensen MC, Brant-Zawadzki MN, Obuchowski N, Modic MT, Malkasian D, Ross JS. Magnetic resonance imaging of the lumbar spine in people without back pain. *N Engl J Med*. 1994;331(2):69–73.

Ji R, Berta T, Nedergaard M. Glia and pain: is chronic pain a gliopathy? *Pain*. 2013;154(1):S10–S28.

Katon W, Sullivan M, Walker E. Medical symptoms without identified pathology: relationship to psychiatric disorders, childhood and adult trauma, and personality traits. *Ann Intern Med*. 2001;134(Suppl Part 2):917–925.

Lang EV, Hatsiopoulou O, Koch T, et al. Can words hurt? Patient–provider interactions during invasive procedures. *Pain*. 2005;114:303–309.

Larauche M, Mulak A, Taché Y. Stress-related alterations of visceral sensation: animal models for irritable bowel syndrome. *J Neurogastroenterol Motil*. 2011;17(3):213–234.

Lewis A. "Psychogenic": a word and it mutations. *Psychol Med*. 1972;2:200–215.

Lutz GK, Butzlaff M, Schultz-Venrath U. Looking back on back pain: trial and error of diagnoses in the 20th century. *Spine*. 2003;28(16):1899–1905.

Mansour AR, Baliki MN, Huang L, et al. Brain white matter structural properties predict transition to chronic pain. *Pain*. 2013;154(10):2160–2168.

Marks EM, Hunter MS. Medically unexplained symptoms: an acceptable term? *Br J Pain*. 2015;9(2):109–114. https://doi.org/10.1177/2049463714535372

McGowan PO, Sasaki A, D'Alessio AC, et al. Epigenetic regulation of the glucocorticoid receptor in human brain associates with childhood abuse, Nat Neurosci, 2009;12:342–348

Melzack R. Phantom limbs, the self and the brain (The D. O. Hebb Memorial Lecture). *Canad Psychol*. 1989;30:1–14.

Melzack R, Casey K. Sensory, motivational, and central control determinants of pain: a new conceptual model. In: Kenshalo D, ed. *The Skin Senses*. Springfield, IL: Thomas; 1968:423–439.

Merskey H. Logic, truth and language in concepts of pain. *Qual Life Res.* 1994(3 Suppl 1):S69–S76.

Merskey H, Bogduk N. eds. *Classification of Chronic Pain.* Seattle, Washington: IASP Press; 1994.

Mika J, Zychowska M, Popiolek-Barczyk K, Rojewska E, Przewlocka B. Importance of glial activation in neuropathic *Eur J Pharmacol.* 2013;716(1–3):106–119.

Mogil JS. The genetic mediation of individual differences in sensitivity to pain and its inhibition. *Nat Acad Sci.* 1999;96(14):7744–7751.

Myers B, Greenwood-Van Meerveld B. Role of anxiety in the pathophysiology of irritable bowel syndrome: importance of the amygdala. *Front Neurosci.* 2009;3:47.

Pain terms: a list with definitions and notes on usage: recommended by the IASP Subcommittee on Taxonomy. *Pain.* 1979;6:247–252.

Price DD. *Psychological Mechanisms of Pain and Analgesia.* Seattle, Washington: IASP Press; 1999.

Price DD. Psychological and neural mechanisms of the affective dimension of pain. *Science.* 2000;288(5472):1769–1772.

Raether M. Psychogene Ischias: über psychogene Ischias-Rheumatismus und Wirbelsäulenerkrankungen: bericht der niederrheinischen Gesellschaft für Naturund Heilkunde in Bonn. *Dtsch Med Wochenschr.* 1917;50.

Raij TT, Numminen J, Närvänen S, Hiltunen J, Hari R. Brain correlates of subjective reality of physically and psychologically induced pain. *Proc Nat Acad Sci U S A.* 2005;102(6):2147–2151.

Richarson RD, Engel CC. Evaluation and management of medically unexplained physical symptoms. *Neurologist.* 2004;10:18–30.

Sawamoto N, Honda M, Okada T, et al. Expectation of pain enhances responses to nonpainful somatosensory stimulation in the anterior cingulate cortex and parietal operculum/posterior insula: an event-related functional magnetic resonance imaging study. *J Neurosci.* 2000;20(19):7438–7445.

Schramme T. On the autonomy of the concept of disease in psychiatry. *Front Psychol.* 2013;4:457.

Schofferman J, Anderson D, Hinds R, Smith G, White A. Childhood psychological trauma correlates with unsuccessful lumbar spine surgery. *Spine.* 1992;17:S1381–S1384.

Stein MB, Koverola C, Hanna C, Torchia MG, McClarty B. Hippocampal volume in women victimized by childhood sexual abuse. *Psychol Med.* 1997;27(4):951–959.

Tracey I. Taking the narrative out of pain: objectifying pain through brain imaging. In: Carr D, Loeser JD Morris DB, eds. *Narrative Pain and Suffering.* Seattle, Washington: IASP Press; 2005:127–163.

Tracey I. Imaging pain. *Brit J Anaesth.* 2008;101:32–39.

van Ravenzwaaij J, olde Hartman TC, van Ravesteijn H, Eveleigh R, van Rijswijk E, Lucassen PLBJ. Explanatory models of medically unexplained symptoms: a qualitative analysis of the literature. *Ment Health Fam Med*. 2010;7:223–231.

Varelmann D, Pancaro C, Cappiello EC, Camann WR. Nocebo-induced hyperalgesia during local anesthetic injection. *Anesth Analg*. 2010;110:868–870.

Wall PD. Three phases of evil: the relation of injury to pain. *Ciba Found Symp*. 1979(69):293–304. https://doi.org/10.1002/9780470720523.ch17

Wallace DJ, Linker-Israeli M, Hallegua D, Silverman S, Silver D, Weisman WH. Cytokines play an aetiopathogenetic role in fibromyalgia: a hypothesis and pilot study. *Rheumatology*. 2001;40:743–749.

Watkins LB, Maier SF. The pain of being sick: implication of immune-to-brain communication for understanding pain. *Annu Rev Psychol*. 2000;51 29–57.

Weissbeckera I, Floyda A, Dederta E, Salmona P, Sephtonb S. Childhood trauma and diurnal cortisol disruption in fibromyalgia syndrome. *Psychoneuroendocrinology*. 2006;31:312–324.

Wurtele SK, Kaplan GM, Keairnes M. Childhood sexual abuse among chronic pain patients. *Clin J Pain*. 1990;6(2):110–113.

Yehuda R, Engel SM, Brand SR, Marcus SM, Berkowitz GS. Transgenerational effects of posttraumatic stress disorder in babies of mothers exposed to the World Trade Center attacks during pregnancy. *J Clin Endocrinol*. 2005;90(7):4115–4118.

Yehuda R, Halligan SI, Bierer LM. Cortisol levels in adult off spring of Holocaust survivors: relation in PTSD symptom severity in the parent and child. *Psychoneuroendocrinology*. 2002;27:171–189.

Zhang T, Meaney MJ. Epigenetics and the environmental regulation of the genome and its function. *Annu Rev Psychol*. 2010;61:439–466.

21 Psychological/Behavioral Therapies

By its very nature, chronic pain is likely to persist to one degree or another. Many patients will be unable to continue their previous work and/or leisure activities. As noted in the previous cases, a variety of maladaptive psychological and behavioral states can emerge. As is the case with many other chronic diseases, those with chronic pain will need to develop as set of coping strategies that allow them to acquire a "new normal," and one that is rewarding. This process will take some time, perhaps three to five years, in significant physical pathology. Medical interventions may provide some symptomatic relief. However, long-term benefit is most probable when the behavioral and psychological aspects can be addressed. Learning to help the patient develop self-help skills and overcome the inevitable psychological barriers is as important as teaching proper nutrition to the patient with diabetes.

This chapter briefly describes various psychological therapies used in the treatment of chronic pain. It focuses heavily on behavioral-based therapies as they are the most researched and often cited. The intent is to provide the clinician with the essential aspect(s) of each therapy. This information can help inform and guide the patient. In addition, there may be elements of these therapies clinicians want to incorporate into their practice. Therefore, when feasible, an illustration is provided as to how to apply a particular therapy. This chapter serves as a reference for the therapies alluded to in the previous case studies.

THERAPIES

Psychodynamic/Insight Therapy

Traditional psychodynamic (psychanalytical) therapy is based of the work of Sigmund Freund. Freud saw the psyche in terms of the workings of the id, ego, and superego. Emotional problems were understood to be a result of inner conflicts between doing what one wants to do (id) and what one needs to do (ego) or should do (superego). The underlying motivational force is the gratification of biologically based instinctual drives. In this context, chronic pain is viewed as a result of the patient being unable to gratify this drive in a socially acceptable manner. Freud theorized that the unconscious "used" the physical insult/injury to stabilize a dynamic conflict created by awareness of repressed urges and to partially gratify drives and conflict via subjective pain, disability, and emotional responses. Freudian psychanalysis generally requires frequent sessions, over a long period, conducted by a therapist with extensive training.

Contemporary psychodynamic therapy, often referred to as insight-oriented psychotherapy, is distinct from psychoanalysis. It is based on the assumptions that (i) there are aspects of our emotional lives of which we are not fully conscious, acting as barriers and limiting our ability to function in a healthy way; (ii) chronic pain is a somatic expression of emotional distress; and (iii) unconscious factors can influence the onset and the maintenance of pain.

Traumatic experiences and the absence of validating responsiveness from those we cared about and depended on are two important events affecting unconscious emotional expectations. The existence of an unconscious mental life is a core assumption of insight-oriented therapy. It is believed that one's problems, symptoms, and general discomforts are rooted in, or caused by, something we are not immediately aware of. The increased incidence of chronic pain among those with a history of childhood emotional, physical, and/or sexual abuse is often alluded to as supporting evidence for this approach.

In a sense, a major goal of insight-oriented therapy is to make the unconscious conscious. The therapy focuses on the patient's self-awareness and understanding of the influence of the past on present behavior. It is emotion-focused and experiential in that it explores ways in which past painful experiences and emotional expectations developed during younger years can contribute to current difficulties (Turk et al, 2008). It is believed that a careful examination of issues that have negatively affected a patient's life will help them to understand and change destructive patterns and feelings. For example, in the case of substance abuse, a psychodynamic/insight approach would encourage the patient to examine unresolved conflicts and symptoms arising from past dysfunctional relationships and which manifest themselves in the need/desire to abuse substances.

Eye Movement Desensitization and Reprocessing

Eye movement desensitization and reprocessing (EMDR) is considered an "integrative, psychotherapeutic approach" involving a desensitization procedure in combination with various interventions designed to develop a more adaptive cognitive and emotional state (Shapiro, 1995). It was initially designed for the treatment of stress- and anxiety-related disorders. However, it has been found to improve coping and reduce chronic pain and suffering. EMDR is said to unlock disturbing memories or beliefs and reprocesses them in a manner so they are no longer disabling. EMDR can be very time-efficient, requiring as few as 3 to 5 hours of treatment. Many potential mechanisms (ie, cognitive, hypnotic, self-disclosure, biological) may account for the effectiveness of EMDR (Grant, 2002).

During EMDR, the patient is instructed to focus on the image, negative cognition, and body sensations while attending to short periods of bilateral stimulation (BLS) known as "sets." BLS can involve eye movements, auditory tones, or tapping. At the end of each set, patients are asked "What do you notice now?" In general, the new material becomes the focus of the next set of BLS. BLS is then used to increase the strength of the positive cognition designated to replace the original negative self-belief and to consolidate the client's cognitive insights (Grant, 2002).

Rhythmic eye movements occurring as part of the EMDR procedure reportedly reduce the intensity of maladaptive thoughts and negative emotions. Indeed, this may have been the reason Freud used a back-and-forth movement of a swing watch to induce a state of hypnosis. Presumably EMDR impacts cortical structures similar to those involved in pain processing (eg, amygdala, hippocampus, and prefrontal cortex [PFC]). A study by Amano and Toichi (2016) compared recall of pleasant memories with and without BLS. BLS subjects demonstrated greater "accessibility" and increased relaxation. Increased activity was noted in the right superior temporal sulcus (STS), and a decrease in the areas of the PFC. The right STS is closely related to memory representation and suggests that BLS may help the recall of more representative pleasant memories, while the PFC is associated with emotional regulation correlating with the subject's feelings of relaxation and emotional comfort.

A systematic review of the literature examined the effects of EMDR on measures of pain intensity, disability, depression, and anxiety (Tesarz et al, 2014). EMDR seemed to have more effect on pain intensity than on anxiety or depression. This seems to support the notions that EMDR impacts pain processing at the cortico-limbic levels, altering the perception of nociceptive information rather than higher brain functions like cognition or coping behavior. It is interesting to note that approaches like cognitive-behavioral therapy (CBT) appear to effect disability and psychological distress more than pain intensity.

Conditioning and Behavioral Therapy

Behavioral therapies are based on empirically derived principles of condition and learning. They are perhaps the most commonly referred approaches in the treatment of chronic pain and have been subjected to rigorous scientific study. The therapies focus on overt behaviors, physiological responses, and cognitive processes. They have proven to be effective at reducing pain ratings, improving coping skills, decreasing disability, improving overall quality of life, and reducing reliance on medications.

The role of conditioning and learning is emphasized in the following statements: "The persistence of both inflammatory and neuropathic pain can only be explained when learning processes are taken into account in addition to sensitization mechanisms" and "Learning process, such as classical and operant conditioning, create memories for pain that are based on altered synaptic connections in supraspinal structures and persist without peripheral input" (Birbaumer and Flor, 1997, p. 441). Most recognize that overt behaviors can be conditioned by the use of various positive and negative reinforcement strategies. The role conditioning plays in neurophysiological processes is often overlooked.

The two basic forms of conditioning are operant and respondent (classical) conditioning. Operant conditioning emphasizes the relationship between antecedent cues and behaviors and consequences. Cues can be external or internal, behaviors can be overt or cognitive, and consequences may be positive or negative. Respondent conditioning is illustrated by the well-known example of associating a ringing bell with food, which, when delivered to a hungry dog, elicits a reflexive salivary response. After a few pairings, the bell alone elicits a similar salivary response. Overt behaviors, thoughts, and neurophysiological responses are all susceptible to conditioning.

The combination of these two conditioning paradigms help to create the placebo effect (Benedetti et al, 2011; Price et al, 2008). As patients experience relief associated with a pill of a specific size, shape, and color, they develop an expectation of relief. An identical pill, even if lacking the essential analgesic agent, is likely to produce at least partial relief. Likewise, the more dissimilar the pill, even if it contains the active ingredient, may be relatively less effective. The same has been demonstrated for negative side effects (ie, nocebo effect; Benedetti et al, 2007 Mondaini et al, 2007). The strength of the conditioned response and the role of expectation is perhaps best illustrated by Kaptchuk et al (2010) when they documented a placebo response even when patients were informed that they were receiving a placebo.

In its most basic form, behavioral therapy can be applied to modifying pain behavior'. Moaning, groaning, posturing, and guarding often become habits that are reinforced by others in the environment. Encouraging loved ones to be more attentive to patients when they are more functional can reduce the frequency of these pain behaviors. Indeed, the presence of a reinforcing (overly attentive) spouse has been shown to increase activity in the emotional areas of the brain, increasing the patient's experience of pain (Flor et al, 1987). Providing verbal reinforcement for increased activity during the clinic visit may counteract the development of a sedentary lifestyle and physical deconditioning, both of which are associated with increased pain and disability. All too often it is the patient's demonstration of, and complaints of, pain that garners all the attention.

In general, pain is thought to emerge from the transmission of information initiated by activation of the peripheral nociceptive system through the dorsal horn of the spinal cord and extending up medial and lateral spinothalamic tracts to various regions of the cortex (Besson, 1999; Tracey and Mantyh, 2007). Research has shown that activity in this pain system can be influenced by unrelated stimuli. For example, one study (Duncan et al, 1987) demonstrated that pairing a light with the onset of a painful stimulus, over time, resulted in the light itself being associated with increased activity in the pain system (ie, conditioned nociception). Clinically, this can be seen when patients begin to experience increased pain even in anticipation of performing an activity previously associated with pain.

This conditioning process, in part, can form the basis for the development of kienisophobia (see Chapter 8). The use of graded exercise therapy or systematic desensitization can be useful (Vlaeyen et al, 2002). In this case, after establishing a baseline level of activity, which the patient can tolerate, they are given of series of small increments (goals) to accomplish (Doleys et al, 1982). They are encouraged not to exceed the assigned goal. This goal-oriented versus pain-oriented approach is very common in physical rehabilitation. Encouragement and reinforcement should accompany improved functioning. This process also helps to reduce pain salience (ie, the meaning and attention given to pain). Patients on a home-based exercise program can be encouraged to simply stand up and march in place during commercials while watching their favorite TV program. Walking 10 minutes after each meal versus trying to do 30 minutes all at once may be more easily tolerated. This simple behavior can help to improve function and control weight as the same time.

Self-Regulation Therapies
Self-regulation can be viewed as the ability to tolerate sensations, situations, and distress by forming appropriate and adaptive responses. Self-regulation therapies assist in the development of skills to aid in the control of emotions, thoughts, physiological responses, and behaviors. Three of the more common procedures include relaxation therapy, biofeedback, and hypnosis. *Relaxation therapy* employs a variety of induction procedures for the purpose of relieving stress, anxiety, general arousal, and pain. Simply encouraging patients to take a deep breath and relax several times a day can be beneficial. A number of books, guides, and tapes are available. Four such techniques are available as YouTube presentations and can be accessed at any time at www.doleysclinic.com.

Biofeedback involves the use of ongoing/real-time feedback of one or more physiological responses for the purpose of helping the patient acquire voluntary control over a particular response. Providing direct feedback along with therapeutic instructions are critical features. Unfortunately, there are therapists that mislead the patient by using relaxation/meditation audios and claiming to be performing biofeedback. Cell phone apps and physiological monitoring devices for home use are readily available. These are best used following some formal instruction. Learning to generalize the self-regulation skills to the real world is an essential aspect of biofeedback. Muscle tension (Schwartz, 2003) and heart rate variability are popular and effective targets (Lehrer and Gevirtz, 2014). Although biofeedback requires sophisticated equipment, DeCharms (2007) has shown that the activity of specific areas of the brain, including those in the pain matrix, can be modified through biofeedback.

Finally, *hypnosis* is an attention-focusing procedure in which changes in a person's behavior or mental state/perception are suggested. It involves deep relaxation and intense concentration. It requires a motivated, imaginative, and trusting patient. Hypnosis has been shown to decrease pain-related affect, decrease pain sensation, and inhibit the transmission of pain impulses at the level of the spinal cord. However, it is important to recognize that some patients can become so focused during an office consultation that they become receptive to new information or ways of thinking (suggestions). Experienced clinicians will recognize and take advantage of this opportunity in engage in cognitive restructuring (CR; see later discussion).

Each of these therapies can also be construed as a type of distraction. Most patients will admit that when occupied mentally or physically, they are less aware of their pain. Thus, the importance of developing new hobbies and interests—a new normal. Too many perseverate on what they cannot do or used to do. They need to get through the grief involved in losing a "life that was" and a "life that was to be" (Doleys, 2014). Some never do, and are destined to live in the past, suffering more depression and pain than necessary.

Cognitively Oriented Therapies

Behavior therapy has been described as coming in three waves: (i) behavior modification and biofeedback based on conditioning and learning theory, as summarized earlier; (ii) CBT; and (iii) mindfulness-based cognitive therapy. CBT focuses on information processing and the introduction of (classical) cognitive therapy popularized by A. Beck (1967, 1979). He believed the key to understanding and solving psychological disturbance lay in consciously identifying and correcting cognitive distortions.

The notion that what we think can influence many aspects of our lives is not new. The Stoic philosopher Seneca (1 BC–65 AD) wrote:

Think your way through difficulties: harsh conditions can be softened, restricted ones can be widened, and heavy ones can weigh less on those who know how to bear them . . . nothing happens to the wise man against his expectation.

Likewise, Epictetus (55–135 BC) noted "Men are disturbed not by things, but by the view which they take of them." Most are familiar with John Milton's observation that "The mind is its own place, and in itself can make a heaven of hell" (*Paradise Lost*, 1667). What psychologists have done is develop a means of precisely identifying these maladaptive and dysfunction cognitions, systematically demonstrated their effect on pain, and created effective and efficient treatments.

Cognitive therapies are based on the assumptions that cognitions/ thoughts can (i) include beliefs, appraisals, attributions, expectations; (ii) effect mood states and overt behavior; (iii) influence our experience of, and reaction to, pain; and (iv) be altered, thus modulating pain in a positive or negative fashion. Cognitive function affects pain in a numbers of ways. *Pain appraisal* is the meaning attached to the pain (ie, expected, accepted, punishment, badge of courage, disease conviction etc.). *Beliefs about pain* regard its impact on disability, function, emotions, need for medication, assistance for others, and control over it. *Coping skills* include such activities as ignoring, relaxing, praying, and distracting, and *self-efficacy* is the belief that they and/or the strategies they apply will be effective.

CBT methodology consists of several steps:

1. Identify maladaptive assumptions, thoughts, ideas, expectations, and attitudes.
2. Use verbal techniques to investigate the reasoning behind specific attitudes and assumptions.
3. Teach the patient to recognize, monitor, and record negative thoughts on a daily record.
4. Help the patient practice more appropriate thoughts, shifting from self-defeating to coping thoughts (Turk, 2002).

TABLE 21.1. **Common Cognitive Distortions**

Cognitive Distortion	Example
Over generalization	"Nobody believes I hurt"
Catastrophizing	"This is driving me insane!!"
Negative predictions	"I doubt that anything will help"
All-or-none	"I can't function with any pain"
Jumping to conclusions	"I will probably get all the complications"
Selective attention	"But I still have a bulging disc"

CR is a core procedure in CBT (see Table 21.1). CR is designed to identify and confront negative thought patterns, some of which appear all but automatic, and help the patient to understand how maladaptive, ineffective, and disruptive they are. Open-ended questions (Socratic questioning), examining the evidence for and against these thoughts (cognitions), generating rational and adaptive alternatives, and rehearsing new ways of thinking and behaving are key aspects of CR. In essence, the goal is to "de-catastrophize" thought patterns (Wright et al, 2017).

Mindfulness-based cognitive therapy (MCBT) combines CBT with mindfulness practices such as meditation and breathing exercises. Mindfulness entails attending to the present moment experience, including thoughts, emotions, and bodily sensations. MCBT teaches attending to mental and physical experiences in a nonjudgmental fashion, as if one is a passive observer—in a sense, awareness without reactivity, that is, being aware of environmental and physiological events while limiting one's emotional reactivity toward them. The two major components are (i) focused awareness (ie, attention regulation) and (ii) open monitoring (ie, affective regulation including emotional nonreactivity and nonjudgmental acceptance; Day, 2017).

Mindfulness is a subtle process that can be difficult to communicate in a traditional office-based practice. It operates in a different way than classic CBT. That is, rather than attempting to alter cognitions by identifying, reality testing, and changing maladaptive, dysfunctional beliefs, the mindfulness concept is based on the idea of acceptance. Cognitions (thoughts) are not viewed as maladaptive or dysfunctional but as a natural consequence of learned experience. Mindfulness models provide an alternative way of responding. Treatment often involves 8 weekly 2.5-hour sessions with a trained therapist.

Acceptance and commitment therapy (ACT) is one of many forms of CBT. ACT uses acceptance and mindfulness strategies mixed with commitment and behavior-change strategies, to increase psychological flexibility. Six core principles of ACT are listed in Box 21.1.

The goals are to stimulate (i) "activity engagement," defined as the pursuit of life activities regardless of pain; (ii) "pain willingness," or the recognition that avoidance and control are often unworkable methods of adapting to chronic pain; and (iii) "thought control,' or the belief that pain can be controlled or changed by altering one's thought. Finally, patients are encouraged to recognize pain chronicity, that is, that their chronic pain may well persist to one degree or another indefinitely (McCracken et al, 2004, 2014). The basis of ACT lies in the assumption that although we experience mental and physical pain, we can learn ways of living a more meaningful and fulfilling life by altering how we think about pain and act in its presence.

Catastrophizing has garnered a great deal of attention in recent decades. Pain catastrophizing (PC) is characterized by the tendency to magnify the threat value of pain stimulus and to feel helpless in the context of pain and

---

BOX 21.1 Core Principles of ACT

Cognitive diffusion: Learning methods to reduce the tendency to reify thoughts, images, emotions, and memories
  Acceptance: Allowing thoughts to come and go without struggling with them
  Contact with the present moment: Awareness of the here and now, experienced with openness, interest, and receptiveness
  Observing the self: Accessing a transcendent sense of self, a continuity of consciousness which is unchanging
  Values: Discovering what is most important to one's true self
  Committed action: Setting goals according to values and carrying them out responsibly.

---

by a relative inability to inhibit pain-related thoughts in anticipation of, during, or following a painful encounter. PC has been conceptualized as both a trait (dispositional) and a state (situation-specific) variable (Quartana et al, 2009). Essentially PC is an exaggerated negative orientation toward pain. It has three components: (i) rumination: "I can't seem to get it out of my mind"; (ii) magnification: "I become afraid that the pain will get worse"; and (iii) helplessness: "I feel I can't stand it anymore" (Sullivan et al, 2001, 2005).

One end point of cognitive therapies is to instill more adaptive coping strategies (Rosenstiel and Keefe, 1983). Patients may not recognize these as coping strategies (see Table 21.2). To them, thoughts such as "I cannot live with this pain," "I rarely get dressed in the morning because it hurts to move," or "I can hardly think of anything else but my pain" are statements of fact. They will reject making more positive or adaptive statements as simply fooling themselves. One way of making the point is to have them consider a situation is which a child constantly berates their own mathematics skills when preparing for a test at school. Illustrating the negative consequences of such maladaptive self-talk seems easier to comprehend. Although infrequently discussed, a strong religious/spiritual orientation has been shown to be an effective coping mechanism and has been associated with improvement in pain and function. (Koenig, 2012; Ferreira-Valente et al, 2019). In addition, patients have often commented on how

TABLE 21.2. **Common Coping Strategies**

Strategy	Example
Coping self-statement	"I tell myself I can overcome the pain."
Reinterpreting	"I tell myself it doesn't hurt."
Ignoring	"I don't think about the pain."
Increasing activity	"I do something active like household chores or projects."
Diverting attention	"I try to think of something else."
Praying/hoping	"I have faith in doctors that someday there will be a cure for my pain."

distracting and invigorating a new and fulfilling relationship, grandbaby, or pet can be.

There is evidence that, when effective, CBT is associated with changes at higher cortical centers. One study showed a modality-specific effect of CBT on the activity in the frontal cortex, cingulate, and hippocampus when compared to paroxetine (Paxil®) in depressed patients (Goldapple et al, 2004). A study using chronic pain patients demonstrated increased grey matter volume (GM) in bilateral dorsolateral prefrontal, posterior parietal, subgenual anterior cingulate/orbitofrontal, sensorimotor cortices, and hippocampus, along with a reduced GM in the supplementary motor area (Seminowicz et al, 2013). The authors suggested that the findings

> reflect compensatory mechanisms to increase descending modulation of pain or freeing of cognitive resources for cognitive or affective reappraisal of pain and pain-related challenges, while changes in sensory and motor regions reflect adaptive responses to the repetitive input of noxious signals [ie, reduced pain salience]. (p. 8)

When CBT was combined with exercise and compared to elective spinal fusion for pain, the outcomes at 1-year follow-up were comparable (Bronx et al, 2003).

Dialectic behavior therapy (DBT) combines CBT techniques to help patients develop new skills to manage painful emotions and decrease conflict in relationships (Linehan, 2015). DBT focuses on four broad areas. First, mindfulness therapy (as noted earlier) helps one to accept and be present in the current moment. Second, distress tolerance is designed to enhance tolerance of negative emotion, rather than trying to escape from it. Third, emotion regulation aids in the acquisition of strategies to manage and change intense emotions that are causing problems. Fourth, increasing interpersonal effectiveness allows for communication with others in a way that is assertive, maintains self-respect, and strengthens relationships.

DBT was initially developed to treat patients with borderline personality disorder and those who were chronically suicidal. DBT has also been effective in treating patients with depression, drug and alcohol problems, posttraumatic stress disorder, traumatic brain injuries, binge-eating disorder, and mood disorders. DBT help patients to develop skills for managing painful emotions and conflictual relationships. DBT can involve individual and groups sessions. It requires a significant time commitment. It is quite complex and comprehensive.

Very little research has been done on the application on DBT to chronic pain. Linton (2009) published a case study, and Drurich et al (2016) presented a paper demonstrating its potential benefit. It is unclear whether DBT will become a mainstream therapy for chronic pain, as there are other approaches that are less time consuming and therefore more economical.

Although CBT appears to have become the gold standard for pain therapy, the procedure is not standardized. For example, CBT varies in number of sessions and specific techniques. The techniques may include relaxation training, systematic graduated goal setting, behavioral activation, activity pacing, problem-solving training, and/or CR (Ehde et al, 2014). A 2015 review of the literature concluded that CBT, in general, had a mild to moderate effect size. Its most robust effect was on "pain experience, cognitive coping and appraisal (positive coping measures), and reduced behavioural expression of pain" (p. 1). Importantly, there were no documented adverse events (Monticone et al, 2015). Although it may seem odd to consider adverse events/side effects in the context of behavioral and cognitive therapies, medical complications and adverse events substantially increase the risk and cost of medically based therapy and should be a consideration when assessing treatment options.

A primary goal of this book is to aid the primary care clinician in obtaining some additional tools for managing the chronic pain patient in the office setting. Although formal CBT by a trained pain psychologist is desirable, the primary care clinician is in a position to have as great of an effect and on more patients. Box 21.2 lists some key cognitions the clinician may endeavor to instill.

As a means of reinforcing these concepts, efforts should be made to address the 5 *As* of pain management in those patients treated for chronic pain (Table 21.3). This information could easily for the basis for the clinical encounter note. Documenting the impact of treatment on each of these areas provides evidence that the clinician is attending to a variety of outcomes beyond the subjective report of pain.

Pain and physical pathology are not the same, and there is not a 1-1 relationship.

Chronic pain is complex and involves biological, psychological, and social components.

Successful treatment involves an variety of therapies.

Management more so than cure is the goal.

The patient must participate in their care.

There is a limit to the amount and type of medications that can be prescribed.

Motivational Interviewing

Unfortunately, there are a number of barriers to successful CBT therapy. First, there are not very many experienced and trained CBT pain therapists. Second, insurance coverage is often limited as CBT is usually billed on Behavioral Health or Mental-Nervous codes. Third, patients have been indoctrinated to pain as a purely physical symptom requiring medical intervention. And, finally, few patients appear motivated and willing to devote the time necessary for a good outcome.

Motivation is big factor in the success of psychological interventions. The Stages of Change Theory (Miller and Rollinick, 2002; Douaih et al, 2005) is an attempt to identify the patient's commitment to change. It grew out of the addiction treatment literature where, unfortunately, relapses occur with regularity. This theory has been adapted

TABLE 21.3.   **The 5 As**

Goal	How to Measure
Analgesia	Can use verbal report or rating scale
Affect	Observation, patient report, significant others' reports, mood scales
Activities of daily living	Select 3 to 5 activities to be improved
Adverse effects	Checklists, exam, labs
Aberrant drug behaviors	Compliance with the medical agreement/ treatment

TABLE 21.4. **Four Stages of Change**

Stage	Description
Precontemplation	Patient is not considering changing behavior
Contemplation	Changes in behavior are being considered
Action	Active steps are being taken to change behavior
Maintenance	Attempts to maintain those changes are evident

to pain management. There are at least four major stages of change (Table 21.4).

Motivational interviewing (MI) is a technique developed to help assess readiness for change. MI assumes that the patient possesses the skills needed to cope but for some reason(s) seems to lack the motivation to apply them. For example, most patients recognize the importance of exercise, weight control, goal-setting, and so on in their pain management. Yet, they fail to implement even the simplest of instructions. Rather than admonishing the patient, the clinician can take a few minutes to identify and clarify the barriers. During MI the clinician elicits the patient's reasons for not making and maintaining adaptive changes. In some instances the clinician may need to seek out and reinforce "importance statements" (eg, "How beneficial do you think it is to get some exercise on a regular basis?"); probing for self-efficacy statements (eg, "It seems you are aware of the importance of increasing your activity; do you feel like you could do something for 10-minutes each day?") and providing affirmation and support are also important ingredients. Many clinicians have seen the patient who complains bitterly about their pain and poor quality of life. Yet, they appear to lack the motivation to change or seek out therapies that do not require any effort on their part, such as medications.

Making medical-based therapy contingent upon some demonstration of behavioral change and motivation for change can minimize the risk of failed treatment and problematic adverse events. The clinician may be accused of lacking compassion, but this is generally a manipulative tactic on the part of the patient to avoid accepting any responsibility for changing their behavior. Some patients will threaten to, and may indeed, seek out a more accommodating clinician. If so, you can be assured that you have done what you can to help the patient help themselves.

SUMMARY

Every office-based encounter involving a patient with chronic pain will have a psychological component to it by virtue of it being an interaction between two individuals. The astute clinician will seize the opportunity to turn these interactions into a teaching moment. Providing education, guiding functional improvement, and remolding maladaptive thoughts can be accomplished. The continuity of care provided in the primary care setting presents an excellent opportunity to introduce and reinforce change over time.

The participation of a trained pain psychologist can be helpful but is not always practical. In addition, patients often are more receptive to such input form their medical provider. A Vox Podcast in 2017 discussing the notion of pain acceptance brought a swift response from patients interpreting the notion of pain acceptance as tantamount to marginalizing them and their experience of pain. They felt the need to have more pain relief options, doctors who are willing to fight for them, and less stigma against using opioids responsibly. Many asserted they have already been forced, in a sense, by their condition to accept and learn to live with their pain but that should not preclude continued efforts to reduce their pain (https://themighty.com/2017/11/pain-acceptance-patient-response-vox/). There has been a good deal of debate regarding misinterpretations of statement made during this podcast and the reaction of other professionals. Helping patients to understand concepts such as pain acceptance, pain coping, and pain-related suffering is as important as the diabetic appreciating the role of diet and exercise in managing patients' disease.

In an effort to increase access to information related to these patients' concerns, our clinic has created a group-based educational session patients are required to participate in. Informal pre-post testing showed improvement in knowledge, self-efficacy, and acceptance. Patients acquired an understanding of appropriate goals/expectations and their role in their therapy. YouTube presentations have been posted (eg, www.doleyclinic.com) to increase access and control costs. We have also made a series of DVDs that could be shown in the clinic's office or viewed at home by the patient and/or family.

Much of the research on psychological/behavioral therapies in the treatment of chronic pain has been done in the academic setting with non-patients or patient volunteers. It is usually highly structured and time-limited. Participants frequently receive some type of inducement. In a word, it is a select and homogenous population. Certain scientific and research criteria have to be met for the findings to be considered valid and reliable. The scientific theory generated may be sound, but the techniques may need to be modified to suit the clinician, the patients, and the setting. More often than not, it is the principles and not the procedures that are of value. It has been surprising to witness the resilience and adaptiveness of many patients with chronic pain, if one simply "hangs in there" with them. Providing continued support, encouragement, and information can pay big dividends. It may take 3 to 5 years for patients to find a new normal; sadly, some never do.

Pain Psychology for Clinicians (2020) could be considered a companion to this book. It provides numerous examples of patient-clinician dialogue to illustrate how certain behavioral/psychological principles can be employed. Detailed examples of statements, explanations, and responses the clinician may want to consider and how these reflect certain behavioral/psychological principles are given. Including these here would be beyond the scope of this book. Whereas this book addresses "What Do You Do Now?," *Pain Psychology for Clinicians* discusses "How Do You Do It?" and "What Do You Say?"

Further Reading

Amano T, Toichi M. The role of alternation bilateral stimulation is establishing positive cognition in EMDR therapy: A multi-channel near-infrared spectroscopy study. *PLoS One*. 2016;11(10):e0162735.

Beck, AT. *Depression: causes and treatment*. Philadelphia: University of Pennsylvania Press; 1967.

Beck AT, Rush AJ, Shaw BF, Emery G. *Cognitive therapy of depression*. New York, NY: Guildford Press; 1979.

Benedetti F, Carlino E, Pollo A. How placebos change the patient's brain. *Neuropsychopharmacology*. 2011;36:339354.

Benedetti F, Lanotte M, Lopiano L, Colloca L. When words are painful: unraveling the mechanism of the nocebo effect. *Neuroscience*. 2007;147:260–271.

Besson JM. The neurobiology of pain. *Lancet*. 1999;353(9164):1610–1615.

Birbaumer N, Flor H. A leg to stand on; learning creates pain. *Behav Brain Sci.* 1997;20:441–442.

Brox JI, Sorensen R, Friis A, et al. Randomized clinical trial of lumbar instrumented fusion and cognitive intervention and exercises in patients with chronic low back pain and disc degeneration. *Spine.* 2003;28:1913–1921.

Cianfrini L, Richardson, E, Doleys DM. *Pain psychology for clinicians.* New York, NY: Oxford University Press; 2020 (in press).

Day M. *Mindfulness-based cognitive therapy for chronic pain: a clinical manual and guide.* New York, NY: Wiley; 2017.

DeCharms RC, Christoff K, Glover GH, Pauly JM, Whitfield S, Gabrieli JDE. Learned regulation of spatially localized brain activation using real-time fMRI. *Neuroimage.* 2004;21(1):436–443.

Doleys DM. *Understanding and Managing Chronic Pain: A Guide for the Patient and Clinician.* Denver, Colorado: Outskirts Press; 2014.

Doleys DM, Crocker M, Patton D. Response of patients with chronic pain to exercise quotas. *Phys Ther.* 1982;62(8):1111–1114. https://doi.org/10.1093/ptj/62.8.1111

Douaihy A, Jensen MP, Jou RJ. Motivating change in persons with chronic pain. In: McCarberg B and S Passik, eds., *Expert guide to pain management.* Philadelphia, PA: American College of Physicians; 2005:217–231.

Duncan GH, Bushnell MC, Bates R, Dubner R. Task-related responses of monkey medullary dorsal horn neurons. *J Neurophysiol.* 1987;57:289–310.

Dyurich A, Prasad V, Prasad AR. *Dialectical behavioral therapy (DBT) as a tool to help manage psychological and emotional aspects of chronic pain.* Paper presented at: AAPM 2016. San Antonio, TX; September 21–25, 2016.

Ehde DM, Dillworth TM, and Turner JA. Cognitive-behavioral therapy for individuals with chronic pain: efficacy, innovations, and directions for research. *Am Psychologist.* 2014;69(2):153–166.

Ferreira-Valente A, Sharma S, Torres S, Smothers Z, Pais-Ribeiro J, Abbott JH, Jensen MP. Does religiosity/spirituality play a role in function, pain-related beliefs, and coping in patients with chronic pain? A systematic review. *J Relig Health.* 2019. doi:10–1007/s10943-019-00914-7

Flor H, Kerns RD, Turk DC. The role of spouse reinforcement, perceived pain, and activity levels of chronic pain patients. *J Psychosom Res.* 1987;31:251–259.

Goldapple K, Segal Z, Garson C, et al. Modulation of cortical-limbic pathways in major depression: treatment-specific effects of cognitive behavior therapy. *Arch Gen Psychiatry.* 2004;61:34–41.

Grant M. EMDR in the treatment of chronic pain. *J Clin Psychol.* 2002;58:150–152.

Kaptchuk TJ, Friedlander E, Kelley JM, et al. Placebos without deception: a randomized controlled trial in irritable bowel syndrome. *PLoS One.* 2010;5:e155591.

Koenig HG. Religion, spirituality, and health: the research and clinical implications. International Scholarly Research Network, Psychiatry. 2012. Article ID 278730, doi:10.5402/2012/278730

Lehrer PM, Gevirtz R. Heart rate variability biofeedback: how and why does it work? *Front Psychol*. 2014;5:756. doi:10.3389/fpsyg.2014.00756

Linehan, M. *DBT skills training manual*. 2nd ed. New York, NY: Guilford Press; 2015.

Linton S. Applying dialectical behavior therapy to chronic pain: a case study. *Scand J Pain*, 31 Dec 2009;1(1):50–54. doi:10.1016/j.sjpain.2009.09.005 PMID: 29913921

McCracken LM, Vowles KE. Acceptance and commitment therapy and mindfulness for chronic. pain: model, process, and progress. *Am Psychologist*. 2014;69:178–187.

McCracken LM, Vowles KE, Eccleston C. Acceptance of chronic pain: component analysis and a revised assessment method. *Pain*. 2004;107:159–166.

Miller WR, Rollinick S. *Motivational interviewing: preparing people to change*. New York, NY: Guilford Press; 2002.

Mondaini N, Gontero P, Giubilei G, Lombardi G, Cai T, Gavazzi A, Bartoletti R. Finasteride 5 mg and sexual side effects: how many of these are related to the nocebo phenomenon? *J Sex Med*. 2007;4:1708–1712.

Monticone M, Cedraschi C, Ambrosini E, et al. Cognitive-behavioural treatment for subacute and chronic neck pain. *Cochrane Database Sys Rev*. 2015;5:CD010664. doi:10.1002/14651858.CD010664.pub2

Price DD, Finniss DG, Benedetti F. A comprehensive review of the placebo effect: recent advances and current thought. *Annu Rev Psychol*. 2008;59:565–590.

Quartana PJ, Campbell CM, Edwards RR. Pain catastrophizing: a critical review. *Expert Rev Neurotherapeutics*. 2009;9(5):745–758. doi:10.1586/ern.09.34

Rosenstiel AK, Keefe FJ. The use of cognitive coping strategies in chronic low back pain patients: relationship to patient characteristics and current adjustment. *Pain*. 1983;17:33–44.

Schwartz M. *Biofeedback: a practitioner's guide*. 3rd ed. New York, NY: Guilford Press; 2003.

Seminowicz DA, Shpaner M, Keaser ML, et al. Cognitive-behavioral therapy increases prefrontal cortex gray matter in patients with chronic pain. *J Pain*. 2013;14(12):1573–1584. doi:10.1016/j.jpain.2013.07.020

Shapiro, F. *Eye movement desensitization and reprocessing: basic principles, protocols, and procedures*. New York, NY: Guilford Press; 1995.

Sullivan MJ, Lynch ME, Clark AJ. Dimensions of catastrophic thinking associated with pain experience and disability in patients with neuropathic pain conditions. *Pain*. 2005;113:310–315.

Sullivan MJ, Thorn B, Haythornthwaite JA, Keefe F, Martin M, Bradley LA, Lefebvre JC. Theoretical perspectives on the relation between pain catastrophizing and pain. *Clin J Pain*. 2001;17:52–64.

Tesarz J, Leisner S, Gerhardt A, Janke S, Seidler GH, Eich W, Hartmann M. Effects of eye movement desensitization and reprocessing (EMDR) treatment in chronic pain patients: a systematic review. *Pain Med*. 2014;15(2):247–263.

Tracey I, Mantyh PW. The cerebral signature for pain perception and its modulation. *Neuron.* 2007;55(3):377–391.

Turk DC, Swanson KS, Tunks ER. Psychological approaches in the treatment of chronic pain patients—when pills, scalpels, and needles are not enough. *Can J Psychiatry.* 2008;53(4):213–223.

Turk D, Gatchel RJ (eds.). *Psychological approaches to pain management: a practitioner's handbook.* New York, NY: Guilford Press; 2002.

Vlaeyen JW, de Jong J, Geilen M, Heuts PH, van Breukelen G. The treatment of fear of movement/(re)injury in chronic low back pain: further evidence on the effectiveness of exposure in vivo. *Clin J Pain.* 2002;18:251–261.

Wright JH, Basco GK, Thase ME, Bosco MR (eds.). *Learning cognitive-behavior therapy: an illustrated guide.* 2nd ed. Washington, DC: American Psychiatric Publishing; 2017.

22 The Psychology of Opioid Tapering

INTRODUCTION

The tapering of opioids has become a new dimension to the opioid crisis/epidemic. The tapering of opioid therapy, independent of whether the goal is reduction or discontinuation, appears to have been more of a psychological and sociological phenomenon than founded on clinical or scientific evidence. A review of the psychological and sociological aspects involved illustrate how, within a couple of decades, the response to a demand for a solution to a problem (ie, the undertreatment of pain) becomes the problem.

This chapter will cover three aspects of opioid tapering. First, it will briefly outline the context of opioid tapering and the dilemmas faced by clinicians and patients alike. Next, is a review of some of the approaches to, and psychological issues involved in, the tapering of opioids. Finally, the tapering of opioid therapy is described as involving three processes or stages: pretaper, tapering, and posttaper. Establishing to proper psychological environment and the use of psychological interventions may significantly increase the likelihood of a successful and sustained outcome.

BRIEF HISTORY

The following represents but a few of the potentially influential events in the development of opioid prescribing and tapering trends. This history is important as it illustrates how impactful certain psychological mind sets can be.

In 1980, a one-paragraph editorial in the *New England Journal of Medicine* (Porter, Hershel, 1980) declared addiction to be rare among users of prescribed opioids. This statement was used by the proponents of opioids as a means of dismissing concerns over the prescribing of opioids as promoting the development of addiction. In 1986, Portenoy and Foley (1986) published an article reporting on the effective management of patients with noncancer pain using opioids. This notion was reinforced by a subsequent article by Portenoy (1990). Ronald Melzack (1988), a psychologist and celebrated pain researcher, asserted that the apparent negative attitude toward the use of opioids was misplaced and should be reconsidered. The psychological environment created in the 1980s was fertile ground for the development and marketing of stronger opioids then ever manufactured before—and implied permission to use them.

The opioid use movement was further advanced by emphasizing the patient's right to effective pain control. In April 1999, an Oregon physician was sanctioned by the Oregon Medical Board for underprescribing (http:www.drcnet.org/wol/087.html#undertreatment. Accessed, 12/5/ 19). In his presidential address to the American Pain Society in 1996, neurologist James Campbell declared pain to be the fifth vital sign. In support of the notion of pain as the fifth vital sign, the Joint Commission on Accreditation of Healthcare Organizations (2000) insisted that pain be addressed "to the patient's satisfaction." Gupta et al (2009) stated, "This study provides the evidence needed for hospitals to make pain care a priority and to achieve patient satisfaction throughout the duration of their hospitalization" (p. 157). This is illustrated by the following question that appeared in a survey the Joint Commission on Accreditation of Healthcare Organizations created: "How often did the hospital or provider do everything in their power to control your pain?" The implication, of course, is that the pain experienced by the patient can be controlled by the clinician. Therefore, the patient has the right to expect the clinician to do whatever is necessary to reduce their pain, albeit a subjective phenomenon.

Within two decades, this mandate was withdrawn (Levy et al, 2018). The American Medical Association withdrew its support for pain as the fifth vital sign in 2016 (https://www.painnewsnetwork.org/stories/2016/6/ 23/ama-defends-vital-sign-policy-on-pain. Accessed December, 2019). In fact, the measuring pain as the fifth vital sign did not increase the quality of pain management (Mularski et al, 2006). At about this same time, the reliance on the numerical rating scale (NRS) as a metric in the treatment of pain was not only called into question (Farrar et al, 2001; Sullivan and Ballantyne, 2016) but was identified as a contributing factor to the opioid epidemic: "The root problem may be neither the high risk or the low efficacy of long term opioid therapy but rather an improper focus on reducing pain intensity" (p. 67).

The Centers for Disease Control and Prevention (CDC; 2016) report may have had the greatest psychological and practical impact on opioid prescribing. Although it was to be (i) a guideline, (ii) for the primary care clinicians, and (iii) one that made provision for the legacy patient, it was adopted as the law of the land. Perhaps, more than any other publication, it has been used to set goals for opioid prescribing and to justify tapering, which at times appears to be done indiscriminately. The same psychological environment and fear of sanction and prosecution, which once fueled increased prescribing, now fuels the opposite. Indeed, the threats of costly legal action against the American Pain Society and the American Academy of Pain Management for ostensibly supporting opioid use with chronic pain at least, in part, if not in total, resulted in their being dissolved. Decades of providing important scientific and clinical research/training virtually ignored. Even to today, opioids are the most common pharmaceutical class involved in malpractice claims resulting in up to 1% of claims (Davis et al, 2020).

Finally, there is the separation of chronic cancer-related pain (CCRP) from chronic noncancer-related pain (CNCP). It is hard to find a guideline that limits, or restricts, the use of opioid in the CCRP population, including the cancer survivor. Patients with cancer-related pain and cancer survivors are excluded in the 2016 CDC guidelines (Davis et al, 2020). The use of the term "cancer pain" began to appear in the literature and media in the middle 1970s. Whereas the use of term "noncancer pain" began to occur with greater regularity around 2000. Box 22.1 lists some of attitudes that may have contributed to a more lenient attitude regarding the use of opioid in CCRP.

Historically, the mortality rate for cancer was fairly high, seeming overshadowing any concerns for opioid addiction or abuse. In addition, the emphasis on the psychosocial aspects of CNCP established it as less devastating and more appropriately approached via rehabilitation (Derbyshire, 2005). Somehow, it seemed logical to assume that the pathophysiology of pain was determined by its etiology (ie, tumor or disc). Thus, CNCP came to be viewed as something less than and not serious enough to warrant the use of opioids.

The landscape, however, has changed. Improved therapies are leading to longer life spans and an increased rate of survival—about 45% in 2007 compared to 23% in the 1970s. Even in the case of cancer survivors, the prescribing of opioids appears to be accorded more flexibility then for CNRP (Sutradhar et al, 2017). The rates of persistent opioid use after cancer treatment vary substantially by patient history of opioid use prior to receiving a cancer diagnosis. The persistent posttreatment opioid use rates were lowest for patients who had never used opioids prior to their cancer diagnosis (3.5%) followed by prior intermittent users (15.0%) and prior chronic users (72.2%). The rate of posttreatment diagnoses of opioid abuse or dependence was 2.9%, and opioid-related admissions occurred in 2.1% of patients (Vitzthum et al, 2020), comparable to some estimates for patients with CNRP. It is also worth noting that the evidence of the effectiveness of opioids with CCRP is no greater than for CCRP (Koyyalagunta et al, 2012; Mesgarpour et al, 2014).

Pain, regardless of it origin, can have devastating effects on the entire human organism. In his 1824 book, Jeremy Bentham identified a number of fallacies used in political debates. One such fallacy he describes as the "sham distinction," better known as a "distinction without a difference." This logical fallacy appeals to a distinction between two things that ultimately cannot be explained or defended in a meaningful way. When it comes to CCRP and CNRP pain, one really must question the scientific basis for drawing a distinction. While there may be a linguistic or conceptual difference between the two options, the actual difference it more apparent than real (Peppin and Svhatman, 2016; Argoff, 2013). Indeed, the classification system proposed in 2019 (Treede et al, 2019) de-emphasizes this distinction by subsuming "Chronic Primary Pain" and "Chronic Cancer-Related Pain," under the heading of "Chronic Pain."

This brief discuss was intended to illustrate how psychological/sociological factors (eg, attitudes, biases, etc.) can shape an entire field. A key phrase in opioid tapering should be "patient-centered." There appears to be a need to be cautious about engaging in rule-governed versus "patient-centered" behavior. This is especially true when the rules appear to be forged out of blatant assertion rather than rational, clinical, decision-making informed by the empirical data.

THE CONTEXT

There are a number of factors that have contributed to the psychological environment supporting the shift prescribing to de-prescribing (tapering) of opioids. These include (i) characterizing the current situation as an opioid epidemic, (ii) associating prescription opioids with fatal overdoses, (iii) highlighting the risk of abuse/addiction, (iv) the lack of effectiveness of opioids, and (v) the misapplication of the CDC 2016 report. It can be useful to understand the data relating to the opioid epidemic, which appears to have formed the foundation for the current emphasis on opioid tapering.

The prescribing of opioids for pain reached its zenith in 2012. Although there was a decrease in the prescribing of opioids after this date, the total opioid-related deaths continued to rise (CDC, 2016). Death rates from fentanyl and synthetic opioids have been climbing steadily as about 2013, leveling off about 2015 to 2017 (Guy et al, 2017). Nearly 70% were attributed to heroine and illicit fentanyl from outside the United States. The growing magnitude of illicit fentanyl is highlighted by a recent report from US Customs and Border Protection noting an increased in confiscated fentanyl from international mail from 1,895 pounds to nearly 2,600 pounds from 2018 to 2019. Indeed, grants and cash awards are being offered for the development of new opioid detection systems.

The use of prescription opioids is often associated with fatal opioid-related overdose. One study (Dunn et al, 2010) reported an opioid overdose rate of 0.51% (51/9940), only one overdose of which was fatal. A second

---

BOX 22.1 **Possible Attitudes Associated With a Relaxed Approached to the Use of Opioids**

- Cancer is the most feared disease; anything associated with it (eg, pain) will be the worse of its kind.
- Mortality rates in 1970s approximated 75%; any associated symptom (eg, pain) could be a contributing cause.
- Fear of addiction was of little consequence given the limited life expectancy; provide whatever the patient need to achieve comfort.
- Pathophysiology of CCRP and CNCP are different; CCRP requires more aggressive treatment.

study involving Veterans Administration patients (Bonhert et al, 2011) reported an opioid-related death rate of 0.49% (750/154,684) this included all patients, regardless of any comorbid diagnosis or adjunctive medication (eg, benzodiazepine). While examining the cause of suicide among patients with chronic pain, Petrosky et al (2018) found that 53.6% of suicide decedents died of firearm-related injuries, 47.2% tested positive for benzodiazepines, and only 16.2% were by opioid overdose. Nonopioid-related suicide deaths were increasing over time while those involving opioids remained stable for the 12-year period studied. Males outnumber females 2:1, and the highest incidence was among those over 70 years of age. Another report examined more than 2,900 fatal overdoses in the state of Massachusetts. Only 1.3% of decedents had an active prescription for the opioid detected in their system on the day of their death (Walley et al, 2019).

Two other sentiments that appear to influence the issue of tapering are the risk of abuse/addiction and effectiveness of treatment. The following is a small sampling of research in these areas. A 2016 national survey conducted by the Substance Abuse and Mental Health Services Administration (2016) reported that 2% of those taking prescription opioids, whether obtained legally or illegally, developed a pain reliever use disorder. Among patients with intractable, noncancer pain receiving long-term, high-dose opioids, the addiction rate was less than 1%. Another study (Edlund et al, 2014) examined a database of over 500,000 patients and found that abuse and addiction rates within 18 months of initiating treatment ranged from 0.12% to 6.1%. A 2016 report (Volkow and McLellen, 2016) concluded that in multiple published studies, rates of carefully diagnose addiction to opioid medication averaged less than 8%. When patients with a prior drug abuse and addiction history were excluded, another study found that about 0.19% developed abuse and addiction to prescribed opioids (Burgess et al, 2014). A Cochran review study found signs of addiction in 0.27% of patient on long-term opioid therapy for noncancer pain (Nobel et al, 2010).

The lack of any demonstrated effectiveness of opioids has been another argument used to justify tapering. However, Gudin et al (2017) summarized a systematic review of long-term (6 months or more) opioid therapy for patients with chronic noncancer pain involving articles published up to March, 2016; 70/267 studies, a total of over 19,000 patients met inclusion criteria. The results indicated that (i) among studies ≥12 months, 31 (91%)

reported an improvement in pain of ≥25% from baseline; (ii) study duration (≥6 to <12 months vs. ≥12) had little effect on the proportion of studies demonstrating a ≥25% and ≥50% reduction, and (iii) 41 studies (76%) reported a ≥30% reduction in pain scores. In addition, a 2010 Cochran review (Nobel et al, 2010) of opioids delivered orally, transdermally, or intrathecally reported that all three modes of administration were associated with clinically significant reductions in pain, but the amount of pain relief varied among studies. To be fair, Kissin (2013) presents the opposite view. At times, the effectiveness of the opioid can have has as much, or more, to do with how it is used versus the opioid itself (Doleys, 2017). In fact, patients seen later versus earlier in the day are 17% more likely to get an increase in their prescribed opioid (Neprash and Barnett, 2019). Clinicians' emphasizing an opioid trial, functional improvement, compliance, and adjunctive therapy are likely to have better outcomes.

The CDC report of 2016 punctuated the opioid crises with what has become a call to action on the part of the medical community, government, and insurance companies. Attempts by the CDC to clarify its position and intent (Dowell et al, 2019) as it relates to reducing opioids, especially in the patient with a long history of use (legacy patient) seems to have had very little impact. Forced tapering, which should only be considered under extreme circumstances (eg, the presence of diversion; Davis et al, 2020) has taken on many forms. In some instances the prescribing physicians have simply stopped prescribing. Others have referred patients out of the practice with little provision for opioid management pending finding a new provider. Perhaps mostly commonly, prescribers are utilizing newly developed guidelines to initiate aggressive tapering without providing any education or supportive therapy. Each of these three approaches can have a devastating psychological impact on the patient. In addition, this poses a difficult situation for the clinician who has kindly agreed to take on the patient abandoned by another prescriber.

Although the unfounded emphasis on the NRS as a metric for effective treatment has be revealed as a source of the opioid crises, it, along with the daily morphine milligram equivalent (MME), have become the standard for judging opioid prescribing. Measures of change in function and quality of life appear to remain secondary or, worse, ignored. Indeed, the author spent over two hours with a consulting company engaged to assist a major health care insurance company to address the issue of opioid prescribing. Cases were reviewed, prescribing patterns discussed, and the maximum recommended opioid goal put forth. The functional and psychological well-being of the patient was never addressed.

In the midst of concerns relating to the opioid epidemic, the CDC guidelines, which outline when the prescribing of, or continuation of, opioid therapy for chronic pain is acceptable, are often overlooked:

Determining When to Initiate or Continue Opioids for Chronic Pain: 1. Nonpharmacologic therapy and nonopioid pharmacologic therapy are preferred for chronic pain. Clinicians should consider opioid therapy only if expected benefits for both pain and function are anticipated to outweigh risks to the patient. If opioids are used, they should be combined with nonpharmacologic therapy and nonopioid pharmacologic therapy, as appropriate. (CDC, 2016, p. 8)

The implications are that (i) under certain circumstance, opioids may be an effective therapy, and (ii) opioid therapy need not be limited to patients with cancer-related pain or end-of-life care. Indeed, the author has a patient with remarkable cystic fibrosis who is alive because her opioid therapy allows her to breather relatively pain-free. Her treatment was initiated, and is continued, in conjunction with her pulmonologist, who initially resisted the idea of the use of opioids over concerns for respiratory depression but now supports their use.

As recently as June 18, 2020, the previously discussed observations were confirmed when the American Medical Association

called for CDC to remove arbitrary limits or other restrictions on opioid prescribing given the lack of evidence that these limits have improved outcomes for patients with pain. Rather, they have increased stigma for patients with pain and have resulted in legitimate pain care being denied to patients. "Hard thresholds should never be used. Where such thresholds have been implemented based on the previous CDC Guideline, they should be eliminated. (Madara, cited in American Medical Association, 2020)

PRETAPERING PROCESS

In 2019 the CDC set forth several recommendations as to when opioid tapering should be considered (see Box 22.2). The tapering process should begin by determining why it should be undertaken. There may be cases where the clinician could undertake a trial reduction. That is, a small reduction, perhaps 5% to 10%, should be undertaken to establish and document the effectiveness, or lack thereof, of the therapy, especially on the patient's quality of life. The patient's psychological status needs to be considered. Stress, anxiety, depression, anger, insomnia, irritability, and disorders such as posttraumatic stress disorder may significantly complicate the tapering process and contribute to a protracted abstinence syndrome (PAS; Manhapra et al, 2018; Davis et al, 2020). Furthermore, it is well known, although not always recognized, that opioids can, in fact, help to stabilize certain psychological/psychiatric states (for a summary, see Doleys, 2017). In such cases, tapering may be contraindicated, or specialized psychiatric support may be needed. Patients demonstrating signs of a substance use disorder, comorbid

---

BOX 22.2 **CDC Recommendations**

As of 2019 the CDC recommends tapering of opioids when the patient:

- Requests a dosage reduction.
- Does not have clinically meaningful improvement in pain and function (eg, at least 30% improvement on the 3-item PEG scale, which assess average pain intensity, pain interference with enjoyment of life, and pain interference with general activity level, on 0–10 scales).
- The opioid dosage ≥50 MME/day[a] without benefit or combined with benzodiazepines.
- Shows signs of substance use disorder (eg, work or family problems related to opioid use, difficulty controlling use) are present.
- Experiences overdose or other serious adverse event.
- Presence of early warning signs for possible overdose risk (eg, confusion, sedation, or slurred speech)

[a]See Centers for Disease Control and Pervention. Pocket guide: tapering opioids for chronic pain. https://www.cdc.gov/drugoverdose/pdf/clinical_pocket_guide_tapering-a.pdf. Accessed December 2, 2019.

---

medical conditions, high MME, and/or long-term opioid therapy are likely to require a more individualized, comprehensive, and protracted tapering program. Customary tapering schedules are based primarily on the pharmacological properties of the particular opioid and not the individual circumstance of the patient.

Educating the patient, defining the tapering schedule, outlining the goal (eg, reduction vs. discontinuation), discussing how withdrawal symptoms will be managed, and reviewing alternative pain management strategies should be done in the pretapering phase. Reassure the patient that tapering does not have to mean discontinuing the opioid. If available, invite your patient to have a discussion with a patient you have successfully tapered. Provide educational material the patient can ponder between sessions. Help them to understand that the lack of present harm does not mean lack of risk.

Some patients need the time and opportunity to build in other strategies for living with chronic pain. Cognitive-behavioral therapy, psychological support, individual counseling, etc. should be available. Psychological support can help the patient cope with anxiety that may arise related to the taper, minimize depression, and establish adaptive coping strategies. This support may include cognitive-behavioral therapy, relaxation, 1:1, etc. Education and goal-setting should be done prior tapering, with support during and after, for up to 12 months. Absent access to other professions, the clinician may find it necessary to set aside a period of time to review the patient's progress.

Some efforts have been put forth to examine the mechanism of tapering and how to prepare the patient. A narrative analysis performed by Matthias et al (2017) identified four key themes regarding patient–provider interaction as it relates to opioid tapering: (i) explaining reasons for tapering, (ii) negotiating the tapering plan, (iii) managing difficult conversations, and (iv) assuring patients that they will not be abandoned. These factors illustrate the importance of creating the proper psychological atmosphere within which to undertake tapering. Box 22.3 lists additional recommendations.

Motivational interviewing may uncover patient perceived barriers to reducing opioids. Restructuring their perceptions can facilitate acceptance. Providing a rational as to "Why now?" can remove the view that the clinician is acting a capricious and uncaring manner. No one can, or should, guarantee the patient that they will not experience any withdrawal symptoms, including a temporary increase in pain. Instead, reassure the patient that everything will be done to minimize these symptoms. Patients can be instructed as to what they can do to address these symptoms. Patient are likely to be more cooperative and accepting if they have some degree of control over the rate at which opioids will be reduced. In some instances, it may be appropriate to allow for a return to a higher level of opioids, if tapering reaches a point where it begins to be associated with a deterioration in one's psychological and functional status.

TAPERING PROCESS

Several apaches have been taken to the tapering of opioids. A time based reduction or a transitioning to, and subsequent tapering from, buprenorphine are probably the most common. Detoxification in a hospital setting may appeal to some patients. A 2006 Cochran Review study (Gowing et al, 2010) warned against the use of the once popular rapid detox or ultra-rapid tapering, secondary to a high risk of adverse events and a strong potential for life-threatening side effects. Furthermore, there was a high rate of relapse as no provisions were made for a maintenance program. The data from this approach supported that removing patients with chronic pain from opioids absent psychological/behavior intervention was inadequate, it not inappropriate.

A recent commentary on opioid tapering noted "rapidly decreasing or abruptly discontinuing long-term opioid analgesics can significantly increase the risk of adverse consequences, including opioid-related hospitalizations and emergency department visits" (Dowell et al, 2019, p. 1855). The US Food and Drug Administration has received reports of serious harm in patients who are physically dependent on opioid pain medicines suddenly having these medicines discontinued or the dose rapidly decreased. These include serious withdrawal symptoms, uncontrolled pain, psychological distress, and suicide. The report stated that no standard opioid tapering schedule exists that is suitable for all patients and urged the clinician to create a patient-specific plan to gradually taper the dose of the opioid and ensure ongoing monitoring and support, as needed, to avoid serious withdrawal symptoms, worsening of the patient's pain, or psychological distress" (US Food and Drug Administration, 2019).

At least two studies have been published illustrating opioid tapering programs with a strong emphasis on the role of psychological interventions ranging from the use of self-help books to intensive group meeting. Darnell et al (2018) describe a tapering program that employed a self-help book on opioid tapering along with a gradual reduction in opioid dosage over a four-month period; 52/119 eligible patients completed the program. The mean MME decreased from 228 to 150. The authors strongly cautioned against a forced taper to zero opioid dose indicating that it could "destabilize an individual both medically and psychologically" (p. 708). It was recommended that patients work with their healthcare clinician to slowly reduce their opioid dose over the one-year time frame. If they wish to go slower or pause the taper, they have that control over the process.

Sullivan et al (2017) randomly assigned 35 patient to either a taper support intervention or usual care. The support group had 18-weekly meetings that explored motivation for tapering and introduced pain self-management skills. The initial requirement of a reduction in 50% (or 120 MME) had to be adjusted to 25% to recruit enough patients. Even so, it took three years to enroll 35/144 patients referred to the study; several recanted their approval and refused to taper while in the program. At 34-weeks, the average reduction for the support group was about 52% (207 to 99 MME) and 44% (245 to 138 MME) for the usual care group. They also noted the absence of any significant increase in pain intensity.

It is interesting to note (i) how difficult it was to recruit patients to participate in the previously discussed studies, (ii) the relatively low percentage of completers, and (iii) that even under these circumstance, patients were still averaging over 100 MME. In their systematic review of literature relating to programs designed for the purpose of reducing opioids, Eccleston et al (2017) concluded, "We are unable to reduce our uncertainty around any treatment offered to these people for this purpose" (p. 12).

POSTTAPERING PROCESS

The ease with which some would assert that tapering and/or discontinuation of opioid therapy in the CNCP population as an answer to the opioid crisis betrays their lack of understanding as to the complexity of the issue. It is based on the misplaced assumption that patients are physically and/or psychological dependent on the opioid and that removing it will return them to more normal state. This notion overlooks the complexity of chronic pain and ignores the possible creation of that which it presumes to espouse to improve: dysfunctional and compromised quality of life.

A thorough reading of Manhapra et al (2018) illustrates otherwise. In it the authors describe and discuss four process occurring in response to neuroplastic behavioral changes emerging with repeated use of opioids: (i) opponent effect, (ii) allostatic reset, (iii) affective dynamism and (iv) PAS. These changes make successful tapering of some patients not only difficult but possibly dangerous. In particular, is the potential unmasking of a PAS related to a refractory dependence of opioids (Ballantyne et al, 2019)? Is it characterized by worsening pain associated with "anxiety, depression, sleep disturbances, fatigue, dysphoria (i.e., feeling down or emotionally blunted), irritability, decreased ability to focus, and deficits in executive control" (Ballantyne et al, 2019, p. 6). Critically, this PAS can last for months or longer.

What happens when opioids are discontinued? It is interesting how enthusiastically opioid tapering (deprescribing) has been promoted, absent data as to the consequences. In one study (Goseling et al, 2019), patients expressed several reasons for wanting to reduce opioids including lack of efficacy, impact on quality of life, and concerns about addiction. However, they were equally concerned about inadequate pain management and the impact of stopping opioids on mood. At the completion of the tapering, 50% reported their pain to be better or the same and 47% reported feeling worse pain. A study involving over 500 veterans (McPerson et al, 2018) noted that 54% of patients reported moderate to severe clinical significant pain after tapering. Sturgeon et al (2020) reported that among patients tapered to less than 90 MME, 52.8% reported greater pain, and 23.6% reported reduced pain. Of those who took part in a buprenorphine transition, 41.8% reported increased pain intensity, and 48.8% reported decreased pain after. High level of opioids and co-utilization of benzodiazepines and/or sedative-hypnotics were associated treatment failure and drop-outs. Quality-of-life measures have not been obtained on a consistent basis indicating a continued misplaced admiration for the NRS. Murphy et al (2013) represent the exception. However, patients were tested pre/post a three-week residential program with no follow-up assessment.

Many of the patients continued on opioids, albeit at a lower level. The need to incorporate a posttapering process is highlighted by Manhpra et al (2018), especially for the long-term user of opioids, to address the previously mentioned PAS. Box 22.4 gives some self-help tips that could be useful during and after the tapering process. Depending on the patient's history and pattern of medication use, dependence counseling following the opioid taper may be needed. Joining a local substance misuse support group (eg, Narcotics Anonymous) or services offered through local church/religious organizations can be cost-effective and beneficial. Two studies (Behar, et al, 2020; Coffin et al, 2020) demonstrated that a significant reduction in, or discontinuation of, opioid therapy was associated with nonprescribed

---

BOX 22.4 **Self-Help Tips for the Patient**

- Drink more water or other liquids than usual.
- Eat regular nutritious meals.
- Use deep-breathing and stretching exercises, as instructed.
- Exercise in moderation (eg, walking).
- Do something to relax (eg, practice relaxation techniques, listen to music or read).
- Use distraction (eg, humor, talking to someone with a positive outlook).
- Use positive self-talk. Tell yourself "I can do this" or "This is only temporary."
- Maximize social support.

opioids and illicit drugs, including heroine. Thus, reinforcing is the need for pretapering planning and posttapering management.

Some patients may insist that they can conduct their own tapering. They should be educated about withdrawal symptoms and encouraged to attempt to slowly taper off opiates before discontinuing completely. By virtue of their compulsive nature, individuals with a substance use disorder may find self-regulated tapering all but impossible and tend to relapse early on in the process. It is noteworthy how many patients are able to transition to different or lesser opioid based on changes in insurance coverage (Schatman, & Webster, 2015) with fewer than anticipated problems—thus the importance of motivation.

SUMMARY

There can be little doubt that, no matter how skillful the clinician, some patients will vehemently object to, and resist, any tapering—some, for good reasons. At this juncture there are limited choices. First, thoroughly document your efforts and remind the patient their progress and status will be monitored carefully. Tapering will be initiated, with or without agreement, if it is apparent that there is significant problem with compliance, diversion, or adverse event(s). Second, impose the taper as conservatively as possible. At times, once it is clear that a given treatment path will be taken, patients acquiesce. Third, if you are unconvinced of the medically necessity, indicate that you will maintain the current regimen for a given period of time during which the patient is free to seek another clinician. However, after that period, tapering will be initiated.

What makes tapering (deprescribing) a psychological phenomenon and not a scientific endeavor is that one can find support for whatever position one wants to promote within the literature. And the research literature is given prominence over the clinical experience. The use a high dose of anything is problematic. Presumably, opioids are prescribed in help improve the patient's quality of life. Yet, the NRS and daily MME remain the defining characteristics of treatment success.

It remains important to understand that most patients are innocent victims in this dilemma. For years, they have done what they were told (ie, taking their medicine as prescribed and insisted upon). Likewise, it was not that long ago the clinicians were chastised, and indeed prosecuted, for undertreating pain. This is the epitome of an iatrogenic problem and one that must appear capricious and arbitrary to the patient. One day agencies are calling pain the fifth vital sign, insisting it be addressed to the patients' satisfaction, and the next, retracting this as a mistake and contributor to the opioid epidemic.

In commenting on the response to the 2016 CDC publication, Dowell et al (2019) indicated the need for better evidence to evaluate the benefits and harms regarding opioid prescribing, including when and how to reduce high-dose opioids in patients receiving them long term. They stated that many of the guidelines have been misapplied, causing serious harm to patients with chronic pain. The CDC does not support abrupt tapering or discontinuation of opioid medication. The guideline's recommendation of 90 MME or less was intended only for patients who are starting opioid therapy. "Unfortunately, some policies and practices purportedly derived from the guideline have in fact been inconsistent with, and often go beyond, its recommendations" including "inflexible application of recommended dosage and duration thresholds and policies that encourage hard limits and abrupt tapering of drug dosages, resulting in sudden opioid discontinuation or dismissal of patients from a physician's practice" (p. 1).

This clarification, although welcomed, does not appear to be stemming the tide of states limiting opioids, insurance companies limiting coverage, guideline consultants harassing providers, and various boards/agencies implying the risk of sanctions or restrictions to clinicians who appear noncompliant. The catch phrases of "patient-centered tapering" and "individualized treatment" do not seem to provide a safe harbor. It is left up to the clinician to use the best available data and resources in determining when and how to navigate the process of opioid tapering. Although incorporating psychological/behavioral interventions at the various stages of tapering will not assuage these issues, it will help to ensure a more patient-centered approach to the tapering of opioids.

Further Reading

American Medical Association. AMA urges CDC to revise opioid prescribing guideline. https://www.ama-assn.org/press-center/press-releases/ama-urges-cdc-revise-opioid-prescribing-guideline. Published June 18, 2020. Accessed July 6, 2020.

Argoff C. Cancer vs noncancer pain: TIME to shed the distinction? Medscape. www.medscape.com/viewarticle/807780_4. Published July 23, 2013. Accessed December 23, 2019.

Ballantyne JC, Sullivan MD, Koob GF. Refractory dependence on opioid analgesics. *Pain.* 2019;160:2655–2660.

Behar E, Bagnulo R, Knight K, Santos GM, Coffin PO. "Chasing the pain relief, not the high": experiences managing pain after opioid reductions among patients with HIV and a history of substance use. PLoS ONE. 2020;15(3):e0230408. https://doi.org/10.1371/journal.pone.0230408

Bohnert AS, Valenstein M, Bair MJ, et al. Association between opioid prescribing patterns and opioid overdose-related deaths. Veterans Health Administration (VHA), 2004 through 2008. *JAMA.* 2011;305(13):1315–1321. https://doi.org/10.1001/jama.2011.370

Burgess HJ, Siddiqui A, Burgess FM. Long-term opioid therapy for chronic pain and the risk of opioid addiction. *R I Med J.* 2014;97(10):25–28.

Centers for Disease Control and Prevention. CDC guideline for prescribing opioids for chronic pain—United States, 2016. *MMWR.* 2016;65(1):1–52.

Coffin PO, Rowe C, Oman N, et al. Illicit opioid use following changes in opioids prescribed for chronic non-cancer pain. *PLoS ONE.* 2020;15(5):e0232538. https://doi.org/10.1371/journal.pone.0232538

Darnall BD, Ziadni MS, Stieg RL, Mackey IG, Kao M, Flood P. Patient-centered prescription opioid tapering in community outpatients with chronic pain. *JAMA Intern Med.* 2018;178(5):707–708.

Davis MP, Digwood G, Mehta Z, McPherson ML. Tapering opioids: a comprehensive qualitative review. *Ann Palliat Med.* 2020;9(2):586–610.

Derbyshire SWG. The biopsychosocial model: meaningless catchphrase or fundamental cornerstone? *J Cancer Pain Symp Palliat.* 2005;1(1):79–84.

Doleys, DM. Philosophical issues and psychological factors determining the effectiveness of opioid therapy: a narrative review. *Pain Physician.* 2017;20:e1091–e1105.

Dowell D, Compton WM, Giroir BP. Patient-centered reduction or discontinuation of long-term opioid analgesics: the HHS guide for clinicians. *JAMA.* 2019;322(19):1855–1856.

Dowell D, Haegerich T, Chou R. No shortcuts to safer opioid prescribing. *N Engl J Med.* 2019;380:2285–2287. https://doi.org/10.1056/NEJMp1904190

Dunn KM, Saunders KW, Rutter CM, et al. Overdose and prescribed opioids: associations among chronic non-cancer pain patients. *Ann Intern Med.* 2010;152(2):85–92.

Eccleston C, Fisher E, Thomas KH, et al. Interventions for the reduction of prescribed opioid use in chronic non-cancer pain. *Cochrane Database Syst Rev.* 2017;11:CD010323.

Edlund MJ, Martin BC, Russo JE, Devries A, Braden JB, Sullivan MD. The role of opioid prescription in incident opioid abuse and dependence among individuals with chronic non-cancer pain: the role of opioid prescription. *Clin J Pain*. 2014;30(7):557–564. https://doi.org/10.1097/AJP.0000000000000021

Farrar JT, Young JP, LaMoreaux L, Werth JL, Poole RM. Clinical importance of changes in chronic pain intensity measured on an 11-point numerical pain rating scale. *Pain*. 2001;94(2):149–158.

Guy GP, Zhang K, Bohm MK, et al. Vital signs: changes in opioid prescribing in the United States, 2006–2015. *MMWR*. 2017;66:697–704.

Goesling DeJonckheere M, Pierce J, Williams DA, Brummett CM, Hassett AL, Clauw DJ. Opioid cessation and chronic pain perspectives of former opioid user. *Pain*. 2019;160(5):1131–1145.

Gowing L, Ali R, White J. Opioid antagonists under heavy sedation or anaesthesia for opioid withdrawal. *Cochrane Database Syst Rev*. 2010;1:CD002022.

Gudin J, Nalamachu S, Wallace LE, Matsuno RK, Coplan PM. The long-term analgesic effectiveness of opioid therapy in chronic non-cancer pain patients: a literature review of randomized controlled, open-label, and epidemiologic studies. *Postgrad Med*. 2016;128:34–35. https://doi.org/10.1080/00325481.2016.1224633

Gupta A, Daigle S, Mojica J, Hurley RH. Patient perception of pain care in hospitals in the United States. *J Pain Res*. 2009;2:157–164.

Joint Commission on Accreditation of Healthcare Organizations. *Implementing the New Pain Management Standards*. Oakbrook Terrace, IL: JCAHO; 2000.

Kissin I. Long-term opioid treatment of chronic nonmalignant pain: unproven efficacy and neglected safety? *J Pain Res*. 2013;6:513–529.

Koyyalagunta D, Bruera E, Solanki D, et al. Systematic review of randomized trials on the effectiveness of opioids for cancer pain. *Pain Physician*. 2012;15(3 Suppl):eS39–eS58.

Levy N, Sturgess J, Mills P. "Pain as the fifth vital sign" and dependence on the "numerical pain scale" is being abandoned in the US: Why? *Brit J Anaesthesia*. 2018;120(3):e435–e438. https://doi.org/10.1016/j.bja.2017.11.098

Manhapra A, Arias AA, Ballantyne JC. The conundrum of opioid tapering in long-term opioid therapy for chronic pain: a commentary. *Subst Abuse*. 2018;39(2):152–161. https://doi.org/10.1080/08897077.2017.1381663

Matthias MS, Johnson NL, Shields CG, et al. "I'm not gonna pull the rug out from under you": patient–provider communication about opioid tapering. *J Pain*. 2017;18(11):1365–1373. https://doi.org/10.1016/j.jpain.2017.06.008

McPherson S, Smith CL, Dobscha S, et al. Changes in pain intensity after discontinuation of long-term opioid therapy for chronic noncancer pain. Pain. 2018;159(10):2097–2104.

Melzack R. *Our attitudes toward narcotics are influenced by unfounded prejudice based on street addicts*. Presidential Address, Fifth World Congress of IASP, 1988.

Mendoza M, and Russell HA. Is it time to taper that opioid? (And how best to do it). *J Fam Pract*. 2019;68(6):324–331.

Mesgarpour B, Griebler U, Glechner A, et al. Extended-release opioids in the management of cancer pain: a systematic review of efficacy and safety. *Eur J Pain*. 2014;18(5):605–616.

Mularski RA, White-Chu F, Overbay D, Miller L, Asch SM, Ganzini L. Measuring pain as the 5th vital sign does not improve quality of pain management. *J Gen Intern Med*. 2006;21(6):607–661.

Murphy JL, Clark ME, Banou E. Opioid cessation and multidimensional outcomes after interdisciplinary chronic pain treatment. *Clin J Pain*. 2013;29(2):109–117. https://doi.org/10.1097/AJP.0b013e3182579935

Neprash HT, Barnett ML. Association of primary care clinic appointment time with opioid prescribing. *JAMA Netw Open*. 2019;2:e1910373.

Noble M, Treadwell JR, Tregear SJ, et al. Long-term opioid management for chronic noncancer pain. Cochrane Database Syst Rev 2010;1:CD006605.

Peppin JF, Schatman ME. Terminology of chronic pain: the need to "level the playing field." *J Pain Res*. 2016;9:23–24.

Petrosky E, Harpaz R, Fowler KA, et al. Chronic pain among suicide decedents, 2003 to 2014: findings from the National Violent Death Reporting System. *Ann Intern Med*. 2018;169(7):448–455.

Porter J, Hershel J. Addiction is rare in patients treated with narcotics. *JAMA*. 1980;302(2):123.

Portenoy RK. Chronic opioid therapy in nonmalignant pain. *J Pain Sympt Manage*. 1990; 5(1 Suppl):S46–S62.

Portenoy RK, Foley KM. Chronic use of opioid analgesics in non-malignant pain: report of 38 cases. *Pain*. 1986;25:171–186.

Schatman ME, Webster LR. The health insurance industry: perpetuating the opioid crisis through policies of cost-containment and profitability. *J Pain Res*. 2015; 8:153–158.

Sturgeon JA, Sullivan MD, Parker-Shames S, Tauben D, Coelho P. Outcomes in long-term opioid tapering and buprenorphine transition: A retrospective clinical data analysis, Pain Medicine, 2020; pnaa029, https://doi.org/10.1093/pm/pnaa029

Substance Abuse and Mental Health Services Administration. Results from the 2016 National Survey on Drug Use and Health: detailed tables. https://www.samhsa.gov/data/sites/default/files/NSDUH-DetTabs-2016/NSDUH-DetTabs-2016.htm#tab1-99aon. Published 2016. Accessed December 8, 2019.

Sutrabhar R, Lokku A, Barbera L. Cancer survivorship and opioid prescribing rates: A population-based matched cohort study among individuals with and without a history of cancer. *Cancer*. 2017;123:4286–4293.

Sullivan MD, Ballantyne JC. Must we reduce pain intensity to treat chronic pain? *Pain*. 2016;157:65–69.

Sullivan MD, Turner JA, DiLodovico C, D'Appolonio A, Stephens K, Chan Y. Prescription opioid taper support for outpatients with chronic pain: A randomized controlled trial. *J Pain*. 2017;18(3):308–318. https://doi.org/10.1016/j.jpain.2016.11.003

Treede RD, Rief W, Barke A, et al. Chronic pain as a symptom or a disease: the IASP classification of chronic pain for the International Classification of Diseases (ICD-11). *Pain*. 2019;160(1):19–27.

US Food and Drug Administration. FDA identifies harm reported from sudden discontinuation of opioid pain medicines and requires label changes to guide prescribers on gradual, individualized tapering. https://www.fda.gov/media/122935/download. Published April 9, 2019. Accessed December 2, 2019.

Vitzthum LK, Riviere P, Sheridan P, Nalawade V, Deka R, Furnish T, Mell LK, Rose B, Wallace M, Murphy JD. Predicting persistent opioid use, abuse, and toxicity maong cancer survivors. *Jr National Cancer Institute*. 2020;112(7):720–727.

Volkow ND, McLellan AT. Opioid abuse in chronic pain: misconceptions and mitigation strategies. *N Engl J Med*. 2016;374:1253–1263. https://doi.org/10.1056/NEJMra150777

Walley AY, Bernson D, Larochelle MR, Green TC, Young L, Land T. The contribution of prescribed and illicit opioids to fatal overdoses in Massachusetts, 2013–2015. *Public Health Rep*. 2019;134(6):667–674.

Index

For the benefit of digital users, indexed terms that span two pages (e.g., 52–53) may, on occasion, appear on only one of those pages.

Tables, figures, and boxes are indicated by *t*, *f*, and *b* following the page number.

2-arachidonoylglycerol (2-AG), 166

abandoned patients, 157–62
  assessment, 159–60
  background, 158–59
  case studies, 157
  overview, 162
  treatment, 161–62
aberrant drug behavior, 152–53
abuse, 62*b*, 197, 212
acceptance and commitment therapy
  (ACT), 82–83, 220*b*, 220
acetaminophen, 92
activities of daily living, 10
acupuncture, 93–94
acute management of FD, 57
AD (Alzheimer's disease), 88. *See also*
  dementia
adaptational model, 55
addiction, 62–65, 62*b*. *See also* substance
  use disorder (SUD)
adjunctive therapies, 93–94
AEA (anandamide), 166
affective-perceptual empathy, 139
African Americans, 118–19
Agency for Health Care Policy and
  Research, 159–60
alcohol, 152
allodynia, 72
alprazolam, 128
alternative medicine, 180
Alzheimer's disease (AD), 88. *See also*
  dementia
American Academy of Pain Medicine,
  66, 158
American Geriatrics Society, 92–94

American Medical Association, 232–33,
  238
American Pain Society (APS), 158, 232
American Society for Addiction
  Medicine, 63–65
amphetamines, 151*t*
anandamide (AEA), 166
anesthesia, 32*t*
anger, 135–43
  assessment, 139–40
  background, 136–39
  case study, 135
  overview, 143
  treatment, 141–42
ANP (apparently normal parts), 45–46
anticonvulsants, 93
antidepressants, 91–92
  for dementia, 93
  FDA approved, 13*t*, 13–14
  placebo response vs., 131
  for sleep disorders, 121–22
anti-epileptic drugs, 91–92
antihistamines, 122
antipsychotics, 112–13
anxiety, 22, 196–97
apparently normal parts (ANP), 45–46
APS (American Pain Society), 158, 232
Australian Healthy Eating Quiz, 181
automated dispensers, 91
avoidance. *See* fear-avoidance cycles

Beck Depression Inventory, 11
behavioral therapy, 214–16. *See also*
  psychological therapies
belief, pain, 218
Bentham, Jeremy, 234

benzodiazepines, 23, 41
  increase in prescribing, 129
  for sleep disorders, 120–21
bilateral stimulation (BLS), 213–14
biofeedback, 216–17
blindness, 32*t*
borderline personality disorder
    (BPD), 35–42
  assessment, 39–40
  background, 36–39
  case study, 35
  overview, 41–42
  treatment, 40–41
brain morphology, 21, 200
Briquet's syndrome. *See* somatic symptom
    disorder (SSD)
broad-spectrum hemp extracts, 174
Broggi, Giovanni, 189
buprenorphine, 67–68, 161

Campbell, James, 232
cannabidiol (CBD), 167–68, 171, 174–75
cannabis and cannabinoids, 165–76
  assessment, 170–71
  background, 166–69
  case study, 165, 175–76
  detection window, 152
  false positives for, 151*t*
  for insomnia, 122
  overview, 176
  treatment, 172–75
Carlson, J., 138–39
case studies
  abandoned patients, 157
  anger, 135
  borderline personality disorder
    (BPD), 35
  cannabis and cannabinoids, 165, 175–76
  chemical coping, 127
  conversion disorder (CD), 27
  delusional parasitosis (DP), 107
  dementia, 87
  depression, 9

dissociative identity disorder (DID), 43
factitious disorders (FD), 51
kinesiophobia (KP), 71
malingering (M), 51
nutritional and dietary supplements, 179
pain catastrophizing (PC), 79
posttraumatic stress disorder
    (PTSD), 17
sleep disorders, 117
somatic symptom disorder (SSD), 97
substance use disorder (SUD), 61–68
urine drug screens (UDS), 147
catastrophizing. *See* pain
    catastrophizing (PC)
Caucasians, 118–19
CBD (cannabidiol), 167–68, 171, 174–75
CBT (cognitive-behavioral therapy), 77,
    82–83, 104, 123, 218–19
CCRP (chronic cancer-related
    pain), 233–34
CCs (chemical copers), 130
CD. *See* conversion disorder
Centers for Disease Control and Prevention
    (CDC), 170, 233
  morphine reductions, 141
  opioid tapering recommendations,
    237–38, 239*b*
  substances, testing for, 150
central sleep apnea (CSA), 120
chain of custody (CoC), 149
chemical copers (CCs), 130
chemical coping, 127–33
  assessment, 130
  background, 128–29
  case study, 127
  overview, 132–33
  treatment, 131–32
childhood trauma, 44–45, 197, 212
chronic cancer-related pain
    (CCRP), 233–34
chronic management of FD, 57
chronic noncancer-related pain
    (CNCP), 233–34

chronic pain
  abandoned patients, 157–62
  anger, 135–43
  borderline personality disorder
    (BPD), 35–42
  cannabis and cannabinoids, 165–76
  chemical coping, 127–33
  conversion disorder (CD), 27–34
  delusional parasitosis (DP), 107–14
  dementia, 87–94
  depression, 9–14
  dissociative identity disorder
    (DID), 43–49
  factitious disorders (FD), 51–58
  kinesiophobia (KP), 71–78
  malingering (M), 51–58
  nutritional and dietary
    supplements, 179–85
  pain catastrophizing (PC), 79–85
  posttraumatic stress disorder
    (PTSD), 17–25
  sleep disorders, 117–24
  somatic symptom disorder
    (SSD), 97–104
  substance use disorder (SUD), 61–68
  urine drug screens (UDS), 147–54
Classification of Chronic Pain (Merskey and
  Bogduk), 191–92
CNCP (chronic noncancer-related
  pain), 233–34
CoC (chain of custody), 149
cocaine, 151*t*, 152
Cochran Review study, 236–37, 241
co-consciousness, 44
cognitive-behavioral therapy
  (CBT), 77, 82–83, 104, 123,
  218–19
cognitive-evaluative empathy, 139
cognitively oriented therapies, 217–23
cognitive restructuring, 77
Comley, A. L., 138–39
complementary therapies, 180
compliance, 148

conditioned nociception, 198
conditioning, 73–74, 198, 214–16
confirmatory testing, 148
conscience (superego), 29
contextual basis of pain, 194–202
  brain morphology, 200
  conditioning and learning, 198
  depression, 194–95
  early life stress/anxiety, 196–97
  epigenetics, 198–99
  expectations, 195
  immune system, 199–200
  medically unexplained symptoms, 201–2
  pain catastrophizing (PC), 195–96
  suggestibility, 196
  words and pain rating, 194
Controlled Substances Act (CSA), 158, 166
conversion disorder (CD), 27–34
  assessment, 30–31
  background, 28–30
  case study, 27
  overview, 34
  symptoms, 29*b*
  treatment, 31–34
coping skills, 218, 221*t*, 221–22
Creative Experiences Questionnaire, 47
criminological model, 55
CSA (central sleep apnea), 120
CSA (Controlled Substances Act), 158, 166

DBT (dialectic behavior therapy), 40,
  48, 222–23
DEA (Drug Enforcement Administration),
  66, 150, 158
delta-9 delta tetrahydrocannabinol,
  167, 172–74
delusional parasitosis (DP), 107–14
  assessment, 109–11
  background, 108–9
  case study, 107
  classification and subtypes, 109*b*
  overview, 114
  treatment, 112–13

dementia, 87–94
    assessment, 89, 90*b*
    background, 88–89
    case study, 87
    overview, 94
    treatment, 90–94
DeMeyer, E. J., 138–39
depression, 9–14
    assessment, 11–12
    background, 10–11
    case study, 9
    as contextual basis of pain, 194–95
    overview, 14
    sleep impairment and, 118
    somatic symptom disorder (SSD)
        with, 99
    theories of pain and, 10*b*
    treatment, 12–14
dermatologists, 112
developmental traumas, 197
*Diagnostic and Statistical Manual of Mental
    Disorders*
    borderline personality disorder (BPD),
        36, 37*b*
    conversion disorder (CD) diagnostic
        criteria, 28*b*
    delusional parasitosis (DP), 108
    dissociative identity disorder (DID),
        44*b*, 44–45
    factitious disorders (FD), 52, 53*b*
    malingering (M), 54*b*, 54
    medically unexplained symptoms, 98–99
    medically unexplained symptoms
        (MUS), 201
    psychogenic pain, 191
    substance use disorder (SUD), 63, 64*b*
dialectic behavior therapy (DBT), 40,
    48, 222–23
Diazepam, 151*t*
Dietary Quality Index, 181
dietary supplements. *See* nutritional and
    dietary supplements
direct-to-consumer advertising, 128–29

dispensers, automated, 91
dissociative identity disorder (DID), 43–49
    assessment, 47–48
    background, 44–47
    case study, 43
    overview, 49
    treatment, 48–49
diversion, 62*b*
Doley Clinic, 226
dosing, 92
DP. *See* delusional parasitosis
drug abusers, 137–38
Drug Addiction Treatment Act, 67
Drug Enforcement Administration (DEA),
    66, 150, 158
Ducasse, D., 38
dystonia, 32*t*

early life stress, 196–97
ECS (endocannabinoid system), 166–67
Edwards, Robert R., 80–81
Ekbom's syndrome. *See* delusional
    parasitosis (DP)
elderly persons
    cognitively impaired, pain in, 90*b*
    PTSD in, 20*b*
electroconvulsive therapy, 48
electronic FD, 55
EMDR (eye movement desensitization and
    reprocessing), 48, 213–14
emotional parts (EP), 45–46
empathy, 139
endocannabinoid system (ECS), 166–67
endogenous opioid system, 136, 141
Engle, G. L., 189
Epictetus, 218
epigenetics, 22, 128, 198–99
expectations, 195
eye movement desensitization and
    reprocessing (EMDR), 48, 213–14

factitious disorders (FD), 51–58
    assessment, 55–57, 56*b*

background, 52–55
case study, 51
overview, 58
somatic symptom disorder (SSD)
    vs., 99–100
treatment, 57–58, 58*b*
FDA (Food and Drug Administration),
    128–29, 158, 169
Fear Avoidance Beliefs Questionnaire, 74
fear-avoidance cycles, 21–22, 23. *See also*
    kinesiophobia (KP)
Federation of State Medical Boards, 66, 158
fentanyl, 235
fentanyl citrate, 113
flavonoids, 169
Foley, K. M., 158–59, 231–32
Food and Drug Administration (FDA),
    128–29, 158, 169
forbidden wish (id), 29
formication, 110–11
Frances, Allen, 131
Freud, Sigmund, 190, 211–12
frontotemporal dementia, 88
functional imaging, 29–30

gas chromatography mass spectrometry
    (GCMS), 148, 149–50
genetic perspective, 29
glial cells, 199–200
goal frustration, 136
grief, 12

hallucinatory pain, 196
Harrison Narcotics Tax Act, 158
The Health Effects of Cannabis and
    Cannabinoids, 172, 173*b*
hemp, 167–69, 168*t*, 174
Hemp Farming Act, 168–69
heroin, 151*t*, 235
histrionic personality disorder, 80
homeostenosis, 89
Huntington's disease dementia, 88
hypnosis, 48, 196, 217

hypogonadism, 68
hyposensitization motivational strategy, 113
hypothalamus-pituitary-adrenal (HPA), 21
hysteria. *See* conversion disorder (CD)

IASP (International Association for the
    Study of Pain), 2, 191–92, 203–4
id (forbidden wish), 29
IL (interleukin), 199–200
immune system, 199–200
injustice, perceived, 136
insight therapy, 211–13
insomnia, 118. *See also* sleep disorders
Insomnia Severity Index, 119
interleukin (IL), 199–200
interleukin 6, 136
International Association for the Study of
    Pain (IASP), 2, 191–92, 203–4
isolated cannabinoids, 174

Joint Commission Accreditation of
    Healthcare Organizations, 158, 232

kinesiophobia (KP), 71–78, 216
    assessment, 74
    background, 72–74
    case study, 71
    overview, 78
    treatment, 74–77
Kirsch, I., 131

learning theory, 29, 198, 214
Lepping, P., 113
lidocaine, 93

malingering (M), 51–58
    assessment, 55–57, 56*b*
    background, 52–55
    case study, 51
    overview, 58
    treatment, 57–58, 58*b*
Malnutrition Screening Tool, 181
malpractice, 142

management treatment, 91
marijuana. *See* cannabis and cannabinoids
marketing, television, 128–29
MCBT (mindfulness-based cognitive therapy), 217, 219–20
medically unexplained symptoms (MUS), 201*b*, 201–2
medical records, 55
medication assisted treatments (MATs), 67, 161
melatonin, 122
Melzack, Ronald, 193, 231–32
menopause, 110–11
methadone, 67–68, 93, 151*t*
methamphetamine, 151*t*
MI (motivational interviewing), 224–25, 240–41
milligrams morphine equivalents (MME), 158
Milton, John, 218
mindfulness-based cognitive therapy (MCBT), 217, 219–20
Minnesota Multiphasic Personality Inventory, 11
misuse, 62*b*
mixed sleep apnea, 120
MME (milligrams morphine equivalents), 158
models of pain processing, 193–94
monosymptomatic hypochondriacal psychosis (primary DP), 108
mood disorder, 137–38
Morgellons disease, 108–9. *See also* delusional parasitosis (DP)
morphine, 151*t*
motivational interviewing (MI), 224–25, 240–41
multiple personality disorder (MPD). *See* dissociative identity disorder (DID)
MUS (medically unexplained symptoms), 201*b*, 201–2
muscle relaxers, 91–92

naloxone hydrochloride, 113
naltrexone, 67
Narcan, 68
Narcotics Anonymous, 244–45
National Community Pharmacists Association, 148
negative emotion, 136
neglect, 44–45
nociplastic pain, 204
nonpharmacological therapies, 93–94
nonpossession form of DID, 44
nonsteroidal anti-inflammatory drugs (NSAIDs), 91–92
nonsuicidal self-injurious (NSSI) behavior, 36–39, 41
nontrauma-related model (NT), 45, 46
numerical pain rating (NPR), 74–75
nutritional and dietary supplements, 179–85
    assessment, 181–82
    background, 180–81
    case study, 179
    overview, 184–85
    treatment, 182–84

obstructive sleep apnea (OSA), 120, 122
occupational therapy, 33
olanzapine, 113
online references
    Australian Healthy Eating Quiz, 181
    Doley Clinic, 226
    medical marijuana laws, 170
    Vox Podcast, 226
operant conditioning, 214–15
opioid-induced hyperalgesia, 63
opioids
    benzodiazepines with, 121, 129
    BPD and, 41
    for cognitive impairment, 91–92, 93
    controlling agitation, 137
    inducing depression, 12
    for PTSD, 23–24
opioid tapering, 161–62, 231–46

CDC Pocket Guide, 161
general discussion of, 245–46
history of, 231–34
overview, 231
posttapering process, 243–45
pretapering process, 239–41
process of, 241–43
psychological/sociological
    factors, 235–38
self-help tips for patients, 244*b*
opioid use disorders (OUDs), 62–63
organic DP, 108
OSA (obstructive sleep apnea), 120, 122

pacemakers, 93–94
pain appraisal, 218
Pain as the 5th Vital Sign campaign,
    158–59, 232–33
pain catastrophizing (PC), 73*f*,
    79–85, 220–21
assessment, 81–82
background, 80–81
case study, 79
as contextual basis of pain, 195–96
overview, 84–85
symptoms, 81*b*
treatment, 82–84
Pain Catastrophizing Scale (PCS), 81
pain processing, models of, 193–94
Pain Psychology for Clinicians
    (Cianfrini), 227
paralysis, 32*t*
Parkinson's disease, 88
paroxetine (Paxil), 222
pathogenic model, 55
Patient Health Questionnaire, 11
Patient Health Questionnaire
    Somatic Symptom Severity Scale
    (PHQ-15), 100–1
PC. *See* pain catastrophizing
PCS (Pain Catastrophizing Scale), 81
perceived injustice, 136
perineuronal net (PNN), 22

personality disorders, 36, 137–38, 141
personality trait disturbance, 36
pharmacotherapy, 91, 103–4
Phenobarbitol, 151*t*
PHQ-15 (Patient Health Questionnaire
    Somatic Symptom Severity
    Scale), 100–1
physical abuse, 18–19, 44–45, 197, 212
physical dependence, 62*b*
physical therapy (PT), 33, 82–83,
    93–94
pimozide, 113
placebo effect, 215
plastic surgery, 129
PNN (perineuronal net), 22
point-of-care (POC) testing, 148
Portenoy, R. K., 158–59, 231–32
possession form of DID, 44
posttapering, opioid, 243–45
posttraumatic stress disorder
    (PTSD), 17–25
assessment, 19–22
background, 18–19
case study, 17
causes of, 19*t*
DID as severe form of, 45
epigenetics and, 198
overview, 24–25
symptoms, 18*b*
treatment, 23–24
Prescription Drug Monitoring
    Program, 160
prescription fraud, 53
pretapering, opioid, 239–41
primary DP (monosymptomatic
    hypochondriacal psychosis), 108
proinflammatory substances, 136
pseudoaddiciton, 62*b*
pseudointellectual patients, 139–40
psychiatrists, 112
psychodynamic therapy, 29, 211–13
psychogenic nonepileptic
    seizures, 32*t*

psychogenic pain, 98, 189–205
    contextual basis of pain, 194–202
    general discussion of, 202–5
    history of, 190–93
    models of pain processing, 193–94
    overview, 189–90
psychological factors of opioid
        tapering, 235–38
psychological therapies, 48, 211–27
    cognitively oriented therapies, 217–23
    conditioning and behavioral
        therapy, 214–16
    eye movement desensitization and
        reprocessing (EMDR), 213–14
    general discussion of, 226–27
    motivational interviewing (MI), 224–25
    overview, 211
    psychodynamic/insight therapy, 211–13
    for PTSD, 24t
    self-regulation therapies, 216–17
psychopharamcology, 24t
psychotropic medications, 103–4, 128
PT (physical therapy), 33, 82–83, 93–94
PTSD. See posttraumatic stress disorder

Raether, M., 190–91
recognition treatment, 90–91
reinforcement theory of depression, 194–95
relaxation therapy, 216
resilience, 72, 128
respondent conditioning, 214–15
risperidone, 113

SA (state anger), 136
Sabet, Kevin, 172
salience, 72, 128
secondary DP, 108, 110
second-hand smoke, 152
sedative-hypnotics, 120–21
seizures, psychogenic nonepileptic, 32t
self-efficacy, 218
self-injurious behaviors (SIB), 38
self-mutilation, 108–9

self-regulation therapies, 216–17
Seneca, 218
serotonin-norepinephrine reuptake
        inhibitors, 93
sexual abuse, 18–19, 44–45, 197, 212
SIB (self-injurious behaviors), 38
SIGECAPS, 11, 11b
Silver Sneakers program, 76
sleep apnea, 120
sleep disorders, 117–24
    assessment, 119–20
    background, 118–19
    case study, 117
    overview, 124
    treatment, 120–23
sleep hygiene, 122–23
Smart Approaches to Marijuana group, 172
smoke, second-hand, 152
sociological factors of opioid
        tapering, 235–38
somatic symptom disorder (SSD),
        97–104, 201–2
    assessment, 99–102
    background, 98–99
    case study, 97
    overview, 104
    treatment, 102–4
Somatic Symptom Scale (SSS-8), 100–1
Somatoform Dissociation
        Questionnaire, 47
Spouse/Significant Other PCS, 81
Stages of Change Theory, 224–25
standardized patients, 56–57
state anger (SA), 136
stimulants, 122–23
stimulus control, 122
stress, early life, 196–97
Suboxone, 67, 161
Substance Abuse and Mental Health
        Services Administration, 236
substance use disorder (SUD), 61–68
    assessment, 63–65
    background, 62–63

case study, 61–68
overview, 68
treatment, 65–68
suggestibility, 196
suicide, 11–12, 13–14, 99,
    112–13, 235–36
Sullivan, Michael, 80–81
sundowners syndrome, 89
superego (conscience), 29
syncope, 32t

Tampa Scale for Kinesiophobia, 74
tapering, opioid. See opioid tapering
TCAs (tricyclic antidepressants),
    93, 121–22
teletherapy, 91
television marketing, 128–29
TENS (transcutaneous electrical nerve
    stimulation), 93–94
terpenes, 169
terrors, 44–45
THC (tetrahydrocannabinol), 150–52
theories of pain, depression and, 10b
theory of structural dissociation of
    personality (TSDP), 45–46
tolerance, 62b
topical medications, 93
trait anger-out, 136. See also anger
transcutaneous electrical nerve stimulation
    (TENS), 93–94
trauma, 44–45, 45b, 197, 212
trauma-related model (TR), 45, 46
Traumatic Experiences Checklist, 47
treatment
    abandoned patients, 161–62
    anger, 141–42
    borderline personality disorder
        (BPD), 40–41
    cannabis and cannabinoids, 172–75
    chemical coping, 131–32
    conversion disorder (CD), 31–34

delusional parasitosis (DP), 112–13
dementia, 90–94
depression, 12–14
dissociative identity disorder
    (DID), 48–49
factitious disorders (FD), 57–58, 58b
kinesiophobia (KP), 74–77
malingering (M), 57–58, 58b
nutritional and dietary
    supplements, 182–84
pain catastrophizing (PC), 82–84
posttraumatic stress disorder
    (PTSD), 23–25
sleep disorders, 120–23
somatic symptom disorder (SSD), 102–4
substance use disorder (SUD), 65–68
urine drug screens (UDS), 152–53
tremor, 32t
tricyclic antidepressants (TCAs),
    93, 121–22
trust, 112b, 112, 153, 217
TSDP (theory of structural dissociation of
    personality), 45–46
2-arachidonoylglycerol (2-AG), 166

unconscious emotional expectations, 212
urine drug screens (UDS), 147–54
    assessment, 149–52
    background, 148–49
    case study, 147
    overview, 154
    treatment, 152–53

valerian root, 122
vascular dementia, 88
veterans, 18
Vox Podcast, 224–25

Wernicke-Korsakoff syndrome, 88
words and pain rating, 194
World Health Organization, 148